Sto

HOW TO SAVE YOUR TEETH

The Preventive Approach

HOW TO SAVE YOUR TEETH

The Preventive Approach

HOWARD B. MARSHALL, D.D.S.

EVEREST HOUSE *Publishers, New York*

Library of Congress Cataloging in Publication Data:
Marshall, Howard B.
How to save your teeth
   Bibliography: p. 306
   Includes index
   1. Teeth—Care and hygiene.   2. Dentistry
Popular works.   I. Title
   RK61.M3   617.6'01   79-51197
ISBN: 0-89696-039-0

Copyright © 1980 by Howard B. Marshall, D.D.S.
All Rights Reserved
Published simultaneously in Canada by
Beaverbooks, Pickering, Ontario
Manufactured in the United States of America
Designed by Judith Lerner
First Edition   RRD1080

THIS BOOK IS DEDICATED first and foremost to my lovely wife Cathy. I thank her for her patience, encouragement, self-sacrifice, contributions, and love.

A special thank you to all my patients, whose dental and periodontal condition, and whose many questions, inspired me to write this book.

To Dean D. Walter Cohen, University of Pennsylvania School of Dental Medicine; Dean Emeritus Doctor Henry M. Goldman, Henry M. Goldman School of Graduate Dentistry, Boston University; and Dr. Gerald Kramer, former Professor and Chairman, Dept. of Periodontology, Henry M. Goldman School of Graduate Dentistry, Boston University, for their dedicated examples as teachers and clinicians.

Special appreciation to Dr. Bob Brackett, who showed me, by example, how hard work and intense concentration in the field of periodontics might ultimately yield much better dental health to many people. He sets a marvelous example of dedication to his profession.

Last but not least, thank you to my parents, Leon and Florine, for their sacrifices, without which I could not have been a periodontist.

Contents

ACKNOWLEDGEMENTS 9

INTRODUCTION Why You're Going to Lose Your Teeth
(and What Can Be Done to Stop It) 11

ONE Why You Have Dental Disease 15

TWO How You Can Have Healthy Gum and Bone 36

THREE How You Can Have Strong, Healthy Teeth 63

FOUR The Right Diet for Strong Teeth and Bone 76

FIVE How You Can Get from Birth to Dentures
Without Really Trying! 93

SIX Finding a Good Dentist 110

SEVEN Dental Costs and Why They Vary 117

EIGHT What You Should Know About a Good
Dental Examination 125

NINE How Teeth are Repaired, Including
Full Mouth Reconstruction 135

TEN The Dental Specialties: Why Do You Need
Them and When Do You Use Them? 155

ELEVEN Oh, My Aching Jaw! (The TMJ Syndrome) 231

TWELVE The Most Frequently Asked Dental
Questions—and Answers 238

THIRTEEN Secrets of an Attractive Smile 252

FOURTEEN New Techniques for Pain Control 262

FIFTEEN Dental Emergencies and Special Situations 268

SIXTEEN Dental Insurance: What You Should
Know About it 283

8   CONTENTS

EPILOGUE   Your Dental Future and the Future of Dentistry   296
DIRECTORY   Where to Purchase Your Supplies   301
BIBLIOGRAPHY   306

Acknowledgments

A COMPREHENSIVE BOOK is never the work of one person. There are many people whose advice and counsel were sought during various phases of completing the manuscript. Rather than just list those friends and colleagues who helped me, I wish to identify their field of expertise. They may someday be of direct help to the reader of this book.

PERIODONTICS   For taking the time to read and critique those chapters pertaining to periodontics, I would like to particularly thank Dr. Ted West, Dr. Marvin Rosenberg, Dr. Jay Siebert, Dr. Arnold Ariavdo, and Dr. Joseph Hochberg.

ORTHODONTICS   For manuscript advice and/or photographic help, thanks to Dr. Michael Diamond, Dr. Mel Liefert, Dr. Mark Lemchen, Dr. Gordon Gaynor.

PEDODONTICS   For manuscript critique and helpful suggestions, Dr. David Levine.

IMPLANTOLOGY   For manuscript help and/or photographic help, Dr. Vic Sendax, Dr. Leonard Linkow, Dr. Ken Judi.

RESTORATIVE DENTISTRY   Many dentist friends shared their thoughts and suggestions. Special thanks to Dr. Frank Cellenza, Dr. Alain Roizen, Dr. Burney Croll, Dr. Ronald Maitland, Dr. Irwin Smigel, Dr. Al Carin, Dr. Harold Schwartz, Dr. Harold Linn, Dr. Paul A. Kaufman.

ORAL SURGERY   For help and cooperation on the manuscript, Dr. Jay Goldsmith.

ENDODONTICS   For manuscript critique and helpful suggestions: Dr. Allen Deutsch.

NUTRITION   This topic was most difficult because of the diversity of views. Special thanks to the following for helping me present a balanced picture: Dr. Warren Levin, Dr. Harold Slavkin, Dr. Michael Alfano, Dr. Harold Rosenberg, Dr. Ruth Carol.

INSURANCE   Again, a very difficult chapter to assemble accurately. Special thanks to the following from the insurance field itself: Mr. Charles H. Meyer, Mr. James McDonald, Dr. Bill Downes, Dr. Mel Raskin, Dr. H. Hellman; in the labor field Mr. Henry Foher.

For special help in the area of the TMJ: Dr. Joseph Ellison.

For special photographic assistance: Dr. A. J. Gwinnett, for his marvelous photographs on bacterial plaque.

DENTAL LABORATORIES   For use of their models as well as their advice, Park Dental Studios, Norbert Richter Dental Laboratory.

Special thanks to those of my patients and friends who took time to read parts of the manuscript and give me helpful suggestions: Diane Miller, Milton Pierce, Paul Michael, Sandra Weisband, Josephine Cook, Edith Dryer, Elizabeth Mersey.

It is my sincere hope that this book makes your life easier, healthier, and happier by showing you how you may have a trouble-free mouth.

INTRODUCTION
Why You're Going to Lose Your Teeth (and What Can Be Done to Stop It)

DID YOU KNOW that if you don't read this book, you may lose your teeth? Why? I'll tell you why. Every year thousands of people are having teeth removed that could have been saved. Every year millions of dollars are spent drilling teeth, filling them, pulling them out, and replacing them. Much of the time, cost and pain could have been avoided. Did you know that in the United States 100 million adults have periodontal disease (pyorrhea)? In 32 million, it has reached an advanced stage. According to one study,* as early as age 13, about 80 percent of a large group of American children had gingivitis, considered by many to be the first step toward periodontal breakdown.

"Periodontal disease accounts for the greatest loss of teeth in humans. . . . Results from the last United States National Health Survey (1969) indicate that almost four of every ten children 6 to 11 years old have periodontal disease in some form. This percentage increases with age, so that in the adult age group (18–79 years) almost 74 percent of the population has periodontal disease in one stage of progression or another." (Dept. of Health, Education, and Welfare, 1972, Table II)†

The same wide spread of incidence of decay exists particularly in children and young adults. If no more decay were to occur, it would

* C. D. Marshall-Day; R. G. Stephens, and L. F. Quigley, *Journal of Periodontology* 26 (1955), 185.
† Goldman and Cohen, *Periodontal Therapy*, 6th Ed., C. B. Mosley & Co.

still be impossible to drill and fill all the remaining cavities with the current dental manpower. This dental epidemic may be attacking you. What are you doing at this time to prevent destruction in your own mouth? How can you avoid major costs, time loss, and dental pain? Do you want to have good, sound teeth, healthy gums and bone? Would you like to eliminate bad breath? Yes? Read on!

The very first step you can take to prevent disease is to learn what causes it. Learn what mouth bacteria can really do. Realize that even though dental disease is occurring at a microscopic level, much of it can be prevented by taking only a few minutes a day to hit the agents of disease where it will hurt them. You must learn how diet influences breakdown, and what foods are most destructive.

You must know which foods and vitamins help build tissue resistance, what you should and should not feed your child, and what harmful foods you should stop eating. You can arm yourself to prevent future dental breakdown.

But what if you want to know where you're at now? Better read on and find out what a thorough dental examination consists of, how to choose a dentist, and when to use a specialist. Find out whether your dentist is keeping up, and how to determine, once you're in his office, whether his philosophies are progressive. Learn about a simple home kit to reduce dental disease if directions for its use are followed exactly as described in this book, and coordinate it with the dietary information also presented here.

I am going to try to cover everything you've wanted to know about your mouth, your smile, bad breath, cavities, gum disease, children's dentistry, tooth movement, restorations, replacements, and more. If you are a younger or middle-aged person, with all or most of your teeth, and take the time to learn what is in this book, you may save between $15,000 and $20,000 in the course of your lifetime.*

Let's start on this self-help adventure now. I truly want to help you avoid lots of pain and lost time. I'd like you to keep your teeth as long as possible . . . your entire life!

---

* Based on current costs of full periodontal care and full-mouth rehabilitation, as well as the frequent need to have "re-do" dental work over the years because of decay, root canal problems, or tooth loss that occurs in the unclean, unperiodontally treated mouth.

HOW TO SAVE YOUR TEETH

The Preventive Approach

ONE

Why You Have Dental Disease

INTRODUCTION: DENTAL DISEASE AS A CHAIN REACTION

Just because your mouth doesn't bother you does not mean it's healthy. Since disease in the body starts out on a cellular level, the first breakdown is so small that you don't even know it's happening. Your brain centers tell you something is wrong only after a lot of tissue or structure has been destroyed. Just as people can walk around with cancer for years and not be aware of it, you can be getting breakdown in your gum and supporting bone without knowing it. When your tooth has just a little decay, or yours gums are just slightly inflamed, they don't hurt. Yet, at some stage, you'll feel it. Most people are surprised when the dentist tells them they have a problem. The patient says, "But I don't feel it!" or "How come it doesn't hurt?" Believe me, by the time it hurts, or gums bleed, you are in trouble! Big trouble! One of my patients brought in her husband for a much needed checkup. He hadn't been to a dentist in seven years, since leaving the military. Two teeth had to be extracted, two more required root canals, and he had lost one third of the bone around his teeth. Could all this have been avoided if he w⌐˙ seen earlier? Most likely yes!

The photograph below shows severe bone loss and tooth breakdown in a skull. How did this individual lose the supporting bone around the teeth? Which teeth could still be saved, and which would be hopeless, if this patient were alive?

Because I've spent much of my adult life treating badly broken-

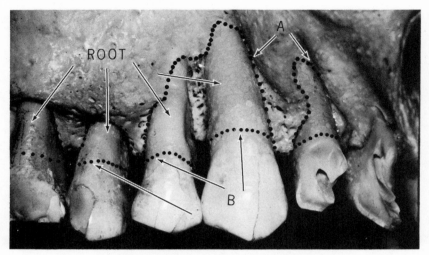

ADVANCED PERIODONTAL DISEASE IN HUMAN SKULL

down mouths, like the one above, and know how much a patient may have to go through, emotionally and financially, to repair the breakdown, I'd like to see you avoid dental pain and large dental costs. I'd rather you not have the mouth like the one shown above. Let's analyze the problem together so you can prevent as much future trouble as possible.

First, let's consider dental disease and see what causes it. We want to know which tissues break down, and why early breakdown, if not corrected, is like a chain reaction. Each untreated problem helps create a bigger problem. The consequences of a chain of dental breakdown are truly amazing:

> 1. The loss of your first permanent molar causes six other teeth to shift, the result of which is a bad bite on that side of your mouth.
> 2. A small cavity, not treated, gets larger, then infects the nerve, causing great pain. To fix the problem may require root-canal work or loss of the tooth.
> 3. Bleeding gums, left untreated, ultimately cause destruction of the underlying bone. This leads to loose teeth and finally tooth loss. Can you imagine biting into an apple and

leaving your tooth in to keep the core company? Or not ever chewing steak or corn on the cob again?

I'm sure that, like most people, you logically assume that if not in pain, your mouth is probably healthy. Not true! Most mouths in the United States and other countries are dentally diseased. Many are at stages where the individual has no pain yet. Often, dental disease may not be recognized very early. Consider yourself fortunate if your dentist has early disease detection and prevention in mind when he examines you.

Dental disease can basically be considered a cause-effect relationship. Bacteria act on your teeth or on your gum and weaken and destroy your enamel or gum tissue. The results of this breakdown in the United States alone are staggering.

Let's look at the following facts:

1. Over 90 percent of Americans are affected by dental disease.
2. The national yearly dental bill is over five billion dollars.
3. It has been estimated that there are 100 million adult Americans with periodontal disease.
4. In one major study, at least 80 percent of children aged thirteen had some degree of gingivitis or inflammation of the gum. This can lead to progressive periodontal disease. "Results from the last United States National Health Survey (1969) indicated that almost four of every ten children 6 to 11 years old have periodontal disease in some form." (Dept. of Health, Education, and Welfare, 1972, Table II)*
5. The transition from gingivitis to periodontitis is evidenced greatly at age fifteen.
6. Periodontal disease is the main cause of tooth loss after age forty. It "is geographically widespread and . . . in most populations, over 50 percent of adults have some form of the

---

* According to another source—*Periodontal Therapy*, Fifth Edition; Goldman & Cohen—between the ages of six and seventeen years, depending on the study, 28 to 64 percent of children were affected by gingivitis. Thus either study indicates a significant percentage of gum disease—gingivitis—in children.

disease." (Dept. of Health, Education, and Welfare, 1972, Table II)

7. Before age 40, decay is the main cause of tooth loss.

8. From the time teeth erupt in the mouth of a baby, they are subject to decay. By age two, approximately 50 percent of America's children have experienced tooth decay.

9. By three years of age, 57 percent of the children have experienced tooth decay.

10. Nearly 50 percent of children under age fifteen have never been to a dentist.

The sad part about these dental problems is that most of them could be prevented.

VARIABLES IN TOOTH BREAKDOWN

Why does all this breakdown occur? Any tissue in the body is a product of its genetic inheritance. But tissues are also influenced by nutrition during formation, and by their environment after formation. The cells of most tissues are constantly metabolizing, frequently regenerating, sometimes dying and being replaced. Nutrition is directly involved in all these reactions because it supplies the essential building blocks of amino acids, vitamins, minerals, and other molecules that permit repair and renewal. This is as true for your gum and bone as for any part of your body. Interestingly, enamel and most of the dentine are unique. They are hard, calcified tissues. Once formed, the original structures do not regenerate, though they may remineralize to a limited degree.

When you think about teeth, gum, and supporting bone, you should be aware of these three areas:

1. Fluoride
2. Diet
   a. The mother's diet during pregnancy
   b. The infant's diet before and after the teeth enter the mouth
3. Oral hygiene

Depending on the interaction of these three variables, the baby's teeth may have average, more, or less resistance to breakdown. In the next chapter, you'll learn about preventing disease, but for the moment let's think about the various causes of dental disease. For example, given a baby whose teeth are showing decay, what factors could cause the decay? For purposes of consideration, let's make four assumptions:

> 1. Assume that the teeth were genetically programmed to form normally.
> 2. Assume that the water fluoridation is adequate (correct range would be 1.0 part per million in a sample of water) and that the baby is getting some of this water.
> 3. Assume that the mother tries to clean the baby's teeth once a day.
> 4. Assume that diet is the only possible cause for breakdown in our example.

If diet is the cause, then as a good detective, you must still raise two questions:

> 1. How did the pregnant mother's diet influence the baby's developing teeth and developing tissue?
> 2. How did the newborn's diet influence the teeth before and after they erupted?

You might also wonder how the diet influences the repair of worn-out structures in the pulp of the tooth, the gum, and the bone throughout your life. We will provide the answers to these questions in Chapters 3 and 4. For the moment, let's examine the tooth itself to see what it's made of, so we will later understand what parts of the tooth break down from disease.

WHAT A HEALTHY TOOTH LOOKS LIKE

To visualize a healthy tooth, look at the cross-section drawing below. The portion of the normal tooth above the gum is called the *crown.* Its covering is a hard substance called *enamel.* Enamel is 97

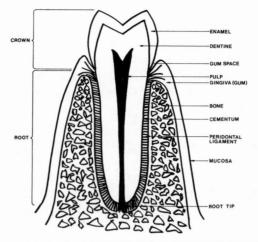

CROWN {

ROOT {

—ENAMEL

—DENTINE

—GUM SPACE

—PULP
—GINGIVA (GUM)

—BONE

—CEMENTUM

—PERIDONTAL
  LIGAMENT

—MUCOSA

—ROOT TIP

CROSS-SECTION OF TOOTH AND SUPPORTING TISSUES

percent mineral, and surrounds the core of the tooth crown. The portion of normal tooth below the gum is called the *root*. It is primarily dentine, covered by a thin layer of tissue called *cementum*. The core is made of *dentine*, both in the crown and in the root. Dentine is 75 percent mineral, the rest being organic material and water. The dentine fills the inside of the tooth, forming most of the bulk of the tooth. It surrounds a "living" tissue, at the center of the tooth, called the *pulp*. You probably know it as the "nerve." The pulp consists of live cells, nerves, and blood vessels which nourish the tooth. It is very fragile and, if injured by decay, or trauma to the tooth, or extremes of cold or hot, the pulp may die. This generally causes you pain and is what you know as a "toothache." A dying or dead nerve can cause one of the most severe pains known to man.

The root of the tooth is covered by a thin, hard material called cementum. The tooth sits in the jawbone, but is separated from it by a ligament called the *periodontal ligament*. The ligament is mainly composed of collagen fibers. The collagen fibers inserting into the cementum help attach the tooth to the surrounding bone. In a normal mouth, where the tooth emerges through the gum, the root stops and the crown begins. The crown is what you see in your mouth, and what you usually call a tooth. Actually, a "tooth" consists of the crown and the root underneath. Remember, the outer layers of the crown are made of enamel, and the material inside is the dentine. Please look carefully at the drawing, and orient yourself to the different tissues of the tooth. The better you remember this drawing, the more easily you'll understand the rest of the dental story.

THE ROLE OF BACTERIA IN DECAY

Without bacteria your teeth would not decay. You have millions of bacteria in your mouth, mainly between your teeth, on your teeth near the gum, and on the tongue. The bacteria have lunch on the food left on the teeth, and like some foods more than others. As bacteria eat and digest the food left on the teeth, they form acids. These acids dissolve the hard mineral surface of your teeth and make holes. We call this process decay. We call the hole a cavity. Lots of holes equal lots of cavities.

The Role of Sugar

People and bacteria have something in common—they both love sweets! Some authorities believe that the worst sugar of all for teeth is sucrose, or ordinary white table sugar. Other authorities feel that glucose or fructose are pretty bad, too. Contrary to some people's belief, brown sugar is just as bad as white sugar. How much importance to give the sugars (glucose, fructose, and sucrose) and refined carbohydrates in causing decay is still not clear to researchers. There are many modifying factors to the sugar-carbohydrate question, including:

1. The chemical structure of the carbohydrate eaten
2. Its consistency (solid, liquid, chewy, sticky, etc.)
3. When it is eaten (i.e., before bedtime, between meals, or with meals)
4. How free the mouth is from bacteria when the food is eaten
5. How soon the mouth is cleansed after eating

In addition, surprisingly small amounts of sugar are all that is needed to offer fermentable food to bacteria. Above those levels, additional carbohydrates or sugars do not seem to change the picture. Thus, in spite of current food fad mythology, the sugar-decay picture is not as simple and clear-cut as one would like.

In spite of this, there are enough scientific papers which have found the role of the "sugars," especially sucrose, to be of concern in causing decay, that it would seem prudent to reduce intake, and restrict it to meal times, until more definite research data is obtained.

It is obvious that sugar is found in many foods, in addition to being eaten in raw form. The table on pages 24–25 can give you an idea of how much sugar is found in some of the common foods you eat. (*Reprinted with permission of the American Dental Association.*)

This table is pretty surprising. There's plenty of sugar in many baby foods, and in many cold cereals. Naturally, there's lots in jelly, jam, pancake syrup, and candy. Sure it tastes good, but what a price the child, or you, may pay in money, time, and maybe pain at the dental office.

Some Important Facts about Bacteria

Let's get back to bacteria, because they are important. There are at least eighty different kinds of bacteria in the mouth, although only three or four are considered most responsible for causing decay. We said that certain bacteria have the ability to break down the sugars into acids. Some bacteria also produce a complicated material called dextran, which is sticky and allows the bacteria to hold tightly to your tooth surface. Other bacteria stick right to the tooth surface itself and work directly on decaying enamel. Still others settle on the backs of the earlier bacterial arrivals.

How do these bacteria, organized in your mouth, do their damage? Basically, they lie in a slimy meshwork composed of several things: saliva, dextran, other bacteria, and food- and salivary-breakdown products. This whole mixture is called plaque. *Plaque (pronounced plak) is the most important word to remember in this book.*

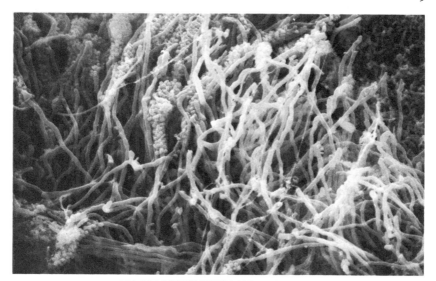

PLAQUE UNDER HIGH MAGNIFICATION

What plaque looks like under the microscope is shown in the illustration above. There are some interesting facts to know about plaque and decay:

1. Studies have shown that *without bacterial plaque*, experimental animals on cavity-prone diets do not develop cavities.
2. Different bacteria are responsible for decay produced in different sites on the tooth.
3. Some bacteria cause decay on the sides of the teeth, some at the gum line, and others on the biting surfaces of the teeth.
4. The bacteria work to destroy the enamel by forming acids.
5. As the acids and the bacteria get deeper into the tooth, different kinds of bacteria actually work together to destroy tooth structure.
6. Bacteria near the tooth surface need oxygen to live.
7. As decay progresses, other bacteria that require less oxygen take over in destroying the tooth.
8. Final result: Your hard tooth has a hole with soft rotting material in it.

FOOD ITEM	SIZE PORTION	APPROXIMATE SUGAR CONTENT IN TEASPOONFUL OF GRANULATED SUGAR
BEVERAGES		
cola drinks	1 (6 oz bottle or glass)	3½
cordials	1 (¾ oz glass)	1½
ginger ale	6 oz	5
highball	1 (6 oz glass)	2½
orangeade	1 (8 oz glass)	5
root beer	1 (10 oz bottle)	4½
Seven-Up*	1 (6 oz bottle or glass)	3¾
soda pop	1 (8 oz bottle)	5
sweet cider	1 cup	6
whiskey sour	1 (3 oz glass)	1½
CAKES AND COOKIES		
angel food	1 (4 oz piece)	7
apple sauce cake	1 (4 oz piece)	5½
banana cake	1 (2 oz piece)	2
cheese cake	1 (4 oz piece)	2
choc. cake (plain)	1 (4 oz piece)	6
choc. cake (iced)	1 (4 oz piece)	10
coffee cake	1 (4 oz piece)	4½
cup cake (iced)	1	6
fruit cake	1 (4 oz piece)	5
jelly roll	1 (2 oz piece)	2½
orange cake	1 (4 oz piece)	4
pound cake	1 (4 oz piece)	5
sponge cake	1 (1 oz piece)	2
canned fruit juices (sweet)	½ cup	2
canned peaches	2 halves and 1 T syrup	3½
fruit salad	½ cup	3½
fruit syrup	2 T	2½
stewed fruits	½ cup	2
DAIRY PRODUCTS		
ice cream	½ pt (3½ oz)	3½
ice cream cone	1	3½
ice cream soda	1	5
ice cream sundae	1	7
malted milk shake	1 (10 oz glass)	5
JAMS AND JELLIES		
apple butter	1 T	1
jelly	1 T	4–6
orange marmalade	1 T	4–6
peach butter	1 T	1
strawberry jam	1 T	4
DESSERTS, MISCELLANEOUS		
apple cobbler	½ cup	3
blueberry cobbler	½ cup	3
custard	½ cup	2
French pastry	1 (4 oz piece)	5
fruit gelatin	½ cup	4½
apple pie	1 slice (average)	7
apricot pie	1 slice	7
berry pie	1 slice	10
butterscotch pie	1 slice	4
cherry pie	1 slice	10
cream pie	1 slice	4
lemon pie	1 slice	7

FOOD ITEM	SIZE PORTION	APPROXIMATE SUGAR CONTENT IN TEASPOONFUL OF GRANULATED SUGAR
brownies (unfrosted)	1 (¾ oz)	3
chocolate cookies	1	1½
Fig Newtons	1	5
gingersnaps	1	3
macaroons	1	6
nut cookies	1	1½
oatmeal cookies	1	2
sugar cookies	1	1½
chocolate eclair	1	7
cream puff	1	2
donut (plain)	1	3
donut (glazed)	1	6
CANDIES		
average choc. milk bar	1 (1½ oz)	2½
chewing gum	1 stick	½
chocolate cream	1 piece	2
butterscotch chew	1 piece	1
chocolate mints	1 piece	2
fudge	1 oz square	4½
gumdrop	1	2
hard candy	4 oz	20
Lifesavers*	1	⅓
peanut brittle	1 oz	3½
CANNED FRUITS AND JUICES		
canned apricots	4 halves and 1 T syrup	3½
mince meat pie	1 slice	4
peach pie	1 slice	7
prune pie	1 slice	6
pumpkin pie	1 slice	5
rhubarb pie	1 slice	4
banana pudding	½ cup	2
bread pudding	½ cup	1½
chocolate pudding	½ cup	4
cornstarch pudding	½ cup	2½
date pudding	½ cup	7
fig pudding	½ cup	7
Grapenut* pudding	½ cup	2
plum pudding	½ cup	4
rice pudding	½ cup	5
tapioca pudding	½ cup	3
berry tart	1 cup	10
blancmange	½ cup	5
brown Betty	½ cup	3
plain pastry	1 (4 oz piece)	3
sherbet	½ cup	9
SYRUPS, SUGARS AND ICINGS		
brown sugar	1 T	*3
chocolate icing	1 oz	5
chocolate sauce	1 T	3½
corn syrup	1 T	*3
granulated sugar	1 T	*3
honey	1 T	*3
Karo syrup	1 T	*3
maple syrup	1 T	*5
molasses	1 T	*3½
white icing	1 oz	*5

* actual sugar content

How Decay Occurs

Now that you understand what a tooth is made of, let's see how decay occurs. We said that bacteria break food products, especially sugars, into acids, which dissolve the enamel crystal. The bacteria themselves produce enzymes, which destroy the cementing material between each crystal. As the enamel dissolves, a hole forms. This hole is called a cavity.

Now what happens? If the cavity is not attended to by removing the decay and filling the hole in the tooth, the decay goes deeper. Up to this point you have not felt pain, because enamel has no nerves. However, once the decay enters the dentine, you may begin to feel slight sensitivity. This sensitivity is caused by stimulation of processes of nerve tissue that come from the pulp.

Early cavities generally don't stimulate the nerve so that your brain realizes something is wrong. Unfortunately, the cavity may have to go very deep toward the nerve (pulp) before you are aware of it. If the cavity is spreading, a strange situation occurs. Though there may only be a small hole or opening at the surface of the tooth, you may have a great deal of decay below the opening, as dental decay has the nasty habit of spreading when it reaches the softer dentine.

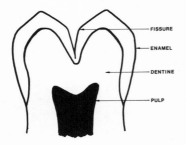

CROSS-SECTION OF CROWN
OF TOOTH SHOWING FISSURES
WHERE DECAY OCCURS

Where Does Decay Occur?

Since there is a definite pattern to the decay of teeth, it is helpful to know on which surfaces of the teeth decay most frequently starts and which teeth are most subject to decay. Decay generally occurs on the biting surfaces of rear teeth that have "tops," or biting

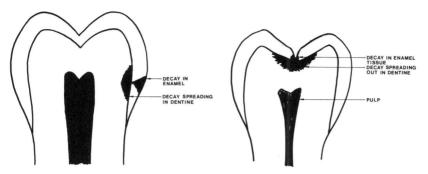

CROSS-SECTION OF CROWN SHOWING
DECAY ON SIDE OF TOOTH

CROSS-SECTION OF CROWN SHOWING
DECAY ON BITING SURFACE OF TOOTH

"tables," as opposed to front teeth, which really have biting "edges." Decay on these rear teeth occurs in the fissures or pits on these "tables." If you look at the teeth in your mouth you'll see lines between solid areas of tooth structure. These are the pits or fissures. In reality, they can run very deeply downward, through the enamel toward the dentine. In cross section, they can look like the illustration above. Beside the tops of the teeth, you can also get decay between teeth, just under the point where the teeth come into contact with each other. Decay occurs in both the pit or fissure, and under the contact point, for two reasons: (1) food and bacteria collect easily there, and (2) they are tough places to reach with a toothbrush.

Lastly, decay can occur on the cheek or tongue side of the tooth next to the gum line. This most frequently occurs if the hygiene is poor. Decay also can occur under an old filling, if it was not well done, or if the original decay was not totally removed. It can also occur if a new filling or gold inlay, onlay, or crown does not have sealed margins or edges where it abuts against the tooth enamel. Because hygiene plays such a major role in preventing decay, you should always brush and floss the entire tooth and gum line daily, remembering that filled or restored teeth are more susceptible to decay than an intact, undrilled tooth. Just because you've had new dental work, don't think that your teeth can't decay again. One of my patients thought that just because she spent a lot of time and money on her teeth, she had done everything necessary to have a healthy mouth. Not true! Poor dental hygiene means dental break-down! Remember, just because a woman spends twenty-five dollars on a facial, that doesn't mean that she never has to wash her face again!

How the Nerve Dies

As the decay gets deeper into the dentine, the gases produced by the dying material and by bacterial products exert pressure on the nerve (pulp). You feel this as a toothache. The pain can be very intense. Remember, the pulp is surrounded on all sides by hard tooth structure. If infected or injured, some pulpal cells start to die, and other cells swell due to inflammation. The buildup of fluid and gases in the pulp can cause swelling, which puts pressure on the tissue at the narrow opening near the root tip. With pressure, the blood supply to the pulp is restricted, or cut off. If this occurs, and the pulp dies, the nerves in the tooth can cause a great deal of pain during the process of self-strangulation.

Saving the Tooth if the Nerve Dies

Do you have to lose your tooth if the nerve dies? The answer is no, whether you're an adult or a child. If a child has a toothache, the tooth may be saved, if not too badly decayed. This is done by taking your child to your dentist, or pedodontist (children's dentist). The tooth is anesthetized (made numb), and the dentist then cleans out the decay and removes the upper portion of the pulp where it enters into the root or roots. The procedure is called a pulpotomy.

When decay has not destroyed too much of the baby tooth, it is important to try to save it. It is important because it helps the permanent tooth to erupt into the proper space. If the tooth were extracted, the remaining teeth might crowd together to fill the space, and thereby block out the permanent tooth. These decisions are made by the dentist or pedodontist. We'll go into this in greater detail in Chapter 9, which covers dental specialties.

Because of anatomical differences in the roots of adult teeth vs. children's teeth, partial removal of the pulp is usually not successful in the adult. With an adult, the entire pulp in the crown and the root is removed to save the tooth. The tooth is filled with a gummy material called gutta-percha, and then protected from fracturing with a crown. This saves the tooth. We'll discuss crowns in Chapters 8 and 10 and go into more detail on root canals in Chapter 9.

THE TOOTH AND ITS SUPPORTING STRUCTURES

So far we have talked about enamel, dentine, pulps, nerves, pulpotomies, and root canals. All this has to do with an individual tooth. But your tooth isn't floating in space. It's held firmly in the jaw and is surrounded at its neck by a collar of gum. Let's examine the anatomy of the gum for a moment, just to understand how gum disease starts around a tooth.

When your tooth erupts into your mouth, it usually grows out of the gum until most or all of its enamel cap is exposed. After eruption, it looks like the illustration below. If we were to very carefully examine the gum area around the neck of the tooth, we could see the following, assuming the gum is healthy.

1. There is a slightly loose collar of gum around the tooth.
2. There is a very tiny space between the gum tissue and the tooth. It's in this space that bacteria live.
3. The gum when we look directly in the front of our teeth rises up and down between each tooth. It should look like an inverted "V" on the upper teeth, or a pyramid on the lower

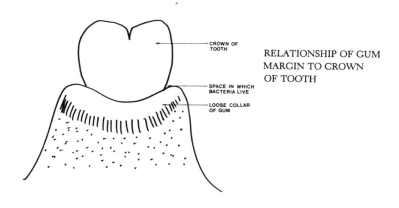

CROWN OF TOOTH

SPACE IN WHICH BACTERIA LIVE

LOOSE COLLAR OF GUM

RELATIONSHIP OF GUM MARGIN TO CROWN OF TOOTH

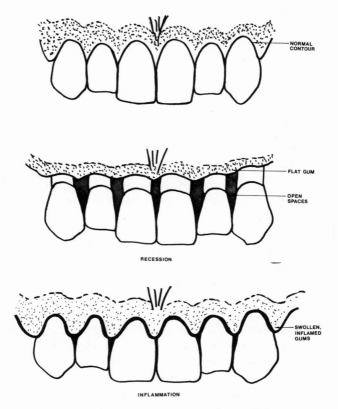

CONTOUR OF NORMAL, RECEDED, AND INFLAMED GUM

teeth. If you have never had periodontal treatment, and your gum is receded, or flattened out between the teeth, with spaces existing between the teeth, you may already have some gum disease. The contour of the healthy gum would look like the illustration above.

4. Where the gum passes on the direct front surface of the upper tooth, the edge may have a little roll, above which is a zone of gum that has a textured, or stippled look. Its appearance in health resembles that of an orange peel. This band of gum is called gingiva. When the gum is inflamed, this textured, stippled effect is lost, and the tissue looks shiny, and swollen.

5. If you pull your upper lip up, you will see that about one-eighth to one-fourth of an inch above the edge, or margin of the gum is a junction running horizontally. Here the textured gum seems to meet another tissue, which is shinier, redder, and through which one may see tiny blood vessels. The first band of tissue described we called gum or gingiva. The shiny tissue is called mucosa. Where they meet is called the mucogingival junction.

HOW GUM DISEASE STARTS

Gingivitis

The space between the gum lining and the tooth is called the *sulcus*. It is critically important because it fills up with bacteria very soon after the tooth erupts. These bacteria, if not removed by brushing and flossing, irritate the gum lining. The bacteria and their products produce an irritation in the lining which causes the lining cells to swell and separate. Then certain enzymes, produced by both the bacteria and the body's cells, destroy the material inside the lining cells, or destroy the cementing substances which hold the cells together. This causes the gum lining to leak inflammatory fluid. Then more bacteria come to live on the leakage products and destroy more tissue. When a sulcus becomes diseased, it is called a *pocket*. A pocket is a space, one side of which is lined by ulcerated gum lining cells and the other side by the tooth.

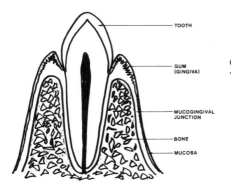

TOOTH

GUM
(GINGIVA)

MUCOGINGIVAL
JUNCTION

BONE

MUCOSA

CROSS-SECTION THROUGH THE
TOOTH, GINGIVA, AND MUCOSA

When this pocket develops, toothbrushing or eating hard foods might cause your gums to bleed. *This bleeding is not normal.* The gum is composed of two tissues: the lining or surface tissue, called *epithelium,* and the dense supportive tissue under it, called *connective tissue.* Certain bacterial enzymes or products, as well as body cells fighting the bacteria, all contribute to further destruction of the connective tissue and its many fiber bundles. A major battle goes on, between the cells your body sends in to fight the bacteria, and other foreign material irritating the gum lining. Although some of the body cells destroy the bacteria, other body cells die in the battle. When these cells die, they release enzymes and other materials which actually destroy more gum tissue and bone. This is a full-scale war! When the bacteria are in the early destruction phase, where the gum lining and the connective tissue are being destroyed, we call this stage *gingivitis.* In your mouth, you can see this stage if your tissue is red, shiny, flabby, or tender, looks slightly puffy or swollen between the teeth, and, frequently, bleeds easily. This stage is produced by bacterial plaque and is reversible.

Periodontitis

The bone that surrounds and supports the tooth begins to be destroyed if the disease goes any deeper. Once bone starts to melt away, the disease is called *periodontal disease,* or *periodontitis.* Pockets are now deeper and contain more bacterial plaque. At this point, the condition is not reversible. Let's repeat that. *Periodontal disease is not reversible.* Now you have a problem. The problem is this: you are irreversibly losing bone! Unfortunately, bone loss causes no pain until very late in the disease. This means that *you could lose more than half your bone* and not know it.

There are some things you might see in looking at your teeth and gums that would indicate possible bone breakdown.

> 1. If the gums are shiny, swollen, or puffy, you may be losing bone underneath.
> 2. If the gums have receded, and there are spaces above where the teeth contact (for upper teeth) and spaces below where the teeth contact (for lower teeth), you probably have lost bone.

3. If you have openings or spaces between teeth that you didn't have as a youngster, you probably have lost bone.

4. Another sign of advancing disease would be tooth looseness.

If you suspect, after examining your gums, that you have a gum problem, start caring more carefully for them. This can be done by brushing and flossing correctly, and using a toothpick in a special way. We'll go into detail on techniques in Chapter 2.

In addition, ask your dentist to "probe" your gums with a *periodontal probe*. This is a small measuring instrument that slips into the gum space between tooth and gum lining. It is marked in millimeters, and as the dentist measures on several sides of the tooth, he can assess how much gum detachment or bone loss has occurred. Probing is essential. *Dental X rays cannot show the amount of bone loss that the probe makes evident.* Every tooth should be measured this way.

One word of warning. If, for any reason, you think the dentist is not familiar with probing, or is being quick and superficial, and too reassuring with statements like "Everything's O.K.—just brush harder," see a periodontist (gum specialist) for a second opinion. You have too much at stake not to protect your gum and bone. Unfortunately, visual and tactile recognition of periodontal breakdown is tricky, and some dentists assume that they are looking at normal tissue when it's really diseased. So if in doubt, a periodontist can help you with an experienced opinion regarding the condition of your gum and bone.

It has been shown without a doubt that gingivitis (gum inflammation) is directly related to poor oral hygiene, and can be reversed by daily removal of plaque. The reason it must be daily (just once) is because the bacteria completely re-form every twenty-four hours. If you let them come back, they'll start destroying again. If plaque is not removed within twenty-four to forty-eight hours, it starts to harden. At that point, you can't

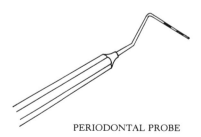

PERIODONTAL PROBE

remove it.

When plaque has hardened and calcified, we call it *calculus* (also called *tartar*). If this hard stuff called tartar or calculus has formed between the teeth, then a dentist or trained dental auxiliary should remove the calculus, and you should continue with daily plaque

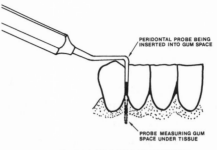

PERIODONTAL PROBE BEING INSERTED INTO GUM SPACE

PROBE MEASURING GUM SPACE UNDER TISSUE

PERIODONTAL PROBE MEASURING A "POCKET"

control (see Chapter 2). If calculus is not removed, it serves as a breeding ground for more bacteria. This leads to more breakdown.

The Cause of Bad Breath

Remember one thing: Plaque doesn't only cause decay and gum disease; it is the primary cause of bad breath. The odor comes from decomposing food and decomposing tissue and bacteria. Bad breath has been blamed on many things, from upset stomachs to garlic, onions, certain cheeses, milk, and smoking. All of these can increase the bad breath *you already have.*

But the single most important cause of bad breath is the garbage on your teeth and in the gum space, and the decomposition of diseased teeth and gum tissue. If you remove plaque once a day, and have decayed teeth cleaned and repaired, most of your bad breath will be eliminated. Get those tender, bleeding gums and gums with periodontal pockets fixed up, and you'll really start to smell kissable. As the advertising industry would say, "Keep the teeth and gums healthy, remove the plaque daily, and you'll be more desirable! Your mouth will feel clean and your breath taste fresh!"

Smoking will make it harder to have clean teeth and nonbleeding gums, because smoke stains leave rough surfaces on the tooth, which bacteria stick to. More bacteria, more odor. If you'd rather not offend anyone after eating, do the plaque control as explained in Chapter 2, and make sure, by being thoroughly examined by a careful dentist, that you have no dental disease. (See Chapter 7.)

Points To Remember

As we said earlier, although gingivitis is reversible, periodontal disease is not. As bone melts away from the gum infection, more bacteria get into the gum space, and more and more destruction occurs. As more bone is lost, the tooth may begin to get loose. At some point, pressures produced by normal chewing my actually rock the tooth in the bone. Continued rocking of the tooth loosens it still further, destroys bone, and may lead to your losing the tooth.

Certain points we have discussed in this chapter are worth repeating:

1. Plaque is the cause of both bacterial decay and gum disease.

2. Plaque must be removed daily to slow or stop disease.

3. Bacteria re-form in twenty-four hours. Therefore, you have to knock them out once every twenty-four hours.

4. With proper mouth hygiene, and tartar removal at the dental office, gingivitis is reversible.

5. Periodontal disease is not reversible, but is treatable. If not treated, you lose bone and later may lose teeth. It is a chronic disease that must be kept in balance by your efforts and periodic visits for professional tartar removal.

The next chapter will discuss how best to clean your mouth and, when repair has to be done, just what parts of your teeth, gum, or bone are being restored or made healthy.

TWO

How You Can Have
Healthy Gum and Bone

MICROSCOPIC BREAKDOWN: THE KEY PROBLEM

If you're not having dental pain, you naturally assume that your mouth is healthy. I'm sure you would think it logical that if something didn't bother you, it must be O.K. Unfortunately, with teeth and gums, that's not the case. As you read earlier, the key problem is that breakdown starts on a tiny, microscopic level. With decay, it starts with bacteria producing acids that dissolve the crystalline portion of a small area of enamel. With gum disease, the bacteria produce reactions in the lining cells of the gum leading to microscopic ulcers. It takes quite a while to get to a stage where you have a toothache, or have your gums bleed.

What can you do to prevent disease from continuing in your own mouth? I use the word "continuing" because everybody has some breakdown occurring on a cellular level. Let's hope it hasn't gotten far enough to cause any real problems.

To start with, let's discuss each area of potential breakdown: 1. the gums; 2. the teeth.

EXAMINATION OF YOUR MOUTH

Necessary Equipment

If your gums and bone aren't healthy, you ultimately won't have any teeth. Suppose we start first with an examination of your gums

36

to see if they're healthy. To do this, I would suggest the following materials:

1. A dental mouth mirror. (You can get this from your drugstore or dentist. See the Directory.)
2. A flashlight.
3. A round mirror, at least five inches in diameter. This five-inch mirror should either come mounted on a stand-up base or, if it is just a plain mirror, be mounted by you in some hard material like plaster or plastic wood. (If you take three strips of cardboard about one and one-half inches high and six inches long and make a triangle, taping the cardboard together, and pour plaster into this, you will have your base and can insert the mirror about one inch into the base.) Now you're ready to examine your mouth.

If you are willing to spend between fifteen dollars and twenty-five dollars, there are two very excellent aids for mouth inspection. One is called the Floxite lamp and the other the Plak-Chek. The Floxite lamp helps you see inside your mouth more clearly because of a strong beam of light and the magnifying mirror into which you look. The Plak-Chek, also an excellent aid, allows you to see the plaque under a special light. The light is blue and the plaque is stained yellow and contrasts easily with your tooth. To stain the plaque with the Plak-Chek setup, you use a yellow disclosing solution. With the Floxite lamp, you use a red tablet or solution. You will have to decide which you prefer, based on discussion with your dentist or pharmacist.

Method of Examination

Using either the Floxite lamp, the Plak-Chek mirror, or resting a flashlight on some books so it will aim directly at the mouth, look in the large round mirror, which is placed about six inches from your mouth. Pull back your lips at the left corner of yor mouth with your fingers. You can retract your lips by holding your left hand with the index finger and middle finger extended, forming an outstretched "V." Fingers should be about one inch apart. The thumb extends

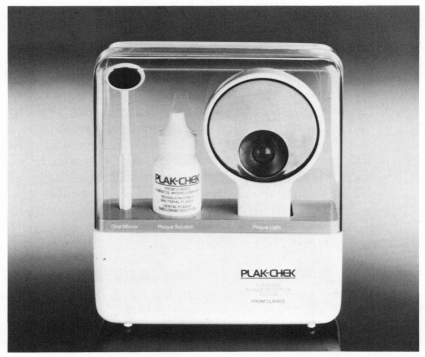

CLAIROL'S "PLAK-CHEK" DISCLOSING LIGHT

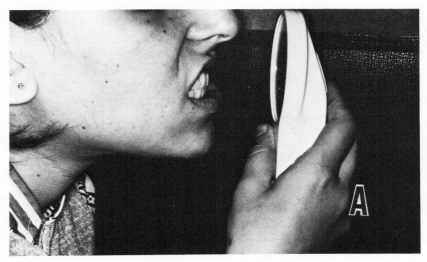

EXAMINING YOUR MOUTH

partially outward in a slightly curved, comfortable position, and the fourth and fifth fingers are curled in to the palm. Open your mouth about one inch, insert the two left fingers, and pull toward that corner of your face. Do the same with the other hand. Now close your teeth—you should look like the illustration on page 38. With the light shining at your gum and with your face about six inches from the mirror, look at your gum and check it.

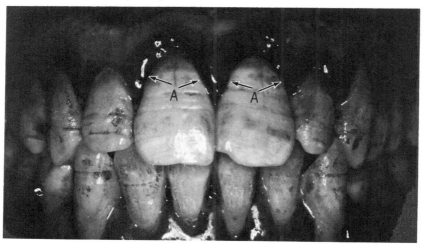

GINGIVITIS (INFLAMED GUM)—ACUTE

Things to Check

1. Is the outline or contour normal?
2. Is the color normal?
3. Is the shape normal?

Let's check each item one at a time.

CONTOUR   Is the contour normal? If healthy, the gum contour will rise up and down between the teeth, in a "V" or cone shape. We call this cone, or pyramid of gum, the *papilla*. If your gum is rounded, or blunt at the tip of the pyramid, it means that there has been recession and loss of bone structure. The only two exceptions to this would be: (1) if your teeth were naturally separated, making your gum flatter; (2) between the rear teeth, where the gum tends to be flatter. The shape is still triangular, but not as high and narrow a triangle as on the front teeth.

Diseased gum generally looks as though someone had removed some tissue from in between the teeth at the gum tip. You would have some space between where the tip of the gum ends and where the teeth meet. Or, your gum could be enlarged and, rather than being pink, might appear slightly red and swollen. Frequently, this happens if you're not into "plaque control." The gum is covered by a collection of food debris and bacterial plaque, which irritates it. The gum swells as it becomes inflamed. Here, too, the contour would not show its usual triangular "rise and fall" shape.

GUM COLOR   Normal, healthy gum is usually pale pink, or coral. It can have degrees of pigmentation. In fact, it can be totally pigmented (brown, bluish brown). This would still be normal as long as shape, contour, and texture are normal. Most people's mouths, if healthy, generally are pink. As your gum gets "sick," irritated by bacterial plaque, it becomes redder, starting with the gum margin. This usually occurs first in the area of the papilla, or tissue triangle between the teeth. Later, it affects the gum right in front of the tooth.

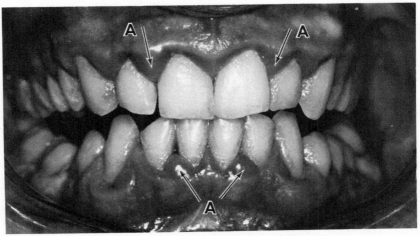

GINGIVITIS (INFLAMED GUM)—CHRONIC

SHAPE   So far we've talked about contour and color. How about the shape of your gum? We said before that the gum in front should look like a pyramid, or cone, in between the teeth. Now look at your gum. Is it flat or thickened between the teeth? Are the tips enlarged? Does it emerge from between the teeth?

This most frequently happens when the gum lining is irritated by bacteria and their products. Your gum responds by overgrowing and enlarging; it is no longer flat, and nicely placed between the teeth, but is bulky and somewhat forward of the teeth. It looks like a swollen, shiny triangle of tissue.

Perhaps your gum has receded and you now have the kind of dark space *between* your teeth that you could enter with a toothpick? If you have a space between your teeth, then your gums may have receded. What about the gum directly on the front of the tooth? Do you see the full crown of enamel? Do you see any more than just the crown? If you can see a darker, yellowish-gray portion of the tooth, you may actually be looking at some root that has been exposed by recession. Since recession may be caused by bad toothbrushing habits, *or* by periodontal disease, you had best be examined by your dentist or periodontist to find our why your root is showing.

Gingivitis

Look at your gum now . . . carefully. See if the gum triangles between the teeth are:

1. Present;
2. If they're pink and normally sized; or
3. If they are enlarged, reddish, and shiny.

If the last, you've got gingivitis (gum inflammation). If that's all that's going on, it's reversible if you follow the plaque-control methods I'll be giving you shortly. If you don't follow the recommendations, you may wind up with bone-destroying periodontal disease.

Also, try pressing on the gum with your fingertip. Look carefully

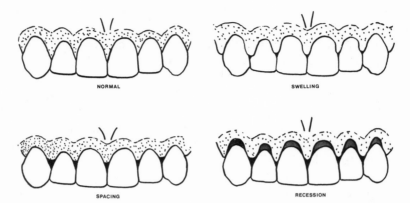

BADLY INFLAMED GUMS WITH HEAVY PLAQUE

and see if a whitish-yellow fluid comes up from the gum space. This is called *exudate*, and is another sign of gum breakdown.

The Periodontal Probe

We must also consider a second possibility. You might have gingivitis *superimposed* on a *chronic periodontal condition*. This can only be established by examining and measuring the gum lining with a fine instrument called a *probe*. This is a most important examination done by your dentist or periodontist. It doesn't hurt at all, and gives tremendous information regarding any gum breakdown or bone loss you may have had. Remember, the big problem in the mouth is that nothing hurts until it's late in the game, so to prevent or treat early, the perio-probe is very important.

We described the probe in Chapter 1; it is a small measuring instrument that slips into the gum space between tooth and gum lining. It is marked in millimeters, and by measuring with it on several sides of the tooth, the dentist can see how much gum detachment or bone loss has occurred. Only your dentist, a periodontist, or a well-trained dental hygienist can examine you with a probe to determine the extent of your gum breakdown. The probe not only reveals how deep the gum space is, but also the quality of the gum lining. Without any pressure, gum lining touched by the probe will bleed if it is broken down and ulcerated. Since the periodontal probing examination is best done in a clean, uninflamed environment anyway, it's still best for you to learn to do the plaque control for several weeks before having your gums measured with the perio-probe. A clean mouth makes for a better exam.

Reversing Gingivitis

If you've been flossing and brushing correctly for several weeks, you will greatly reduce the amount of gum inflammation. The inflamed gum shrinks toward the bone as it gets healthy. So if your gum is getting less red and less inflamed, and is shrinking, that's great. You may be surprised that some spaces are forming between the teeth as the gum shrinks. This is normal and desirable. It means that you are starting to arrest the disease and the swollen, inflamed gum is shrinking toward a more normal size. It's your first big step back toward health.

Let me repeat this important point: *If you have had gum disease for a while, some bone may also have been destroyed under the gum.* As the gum shrinks toward your present bone level, you notice small openings developing between the teeth. This is normal and good. It means that you are reducing the inflammation, and the gum is tightening and moving toward its junction with the bone. Another thing you might notice as inflamed gum shrinks is that a little more of the tooth shows. This is normal and good. You may see some dark brown or green stains on the tooth near the gum. The tooth itself may seem a darker grayish-yellow. This would be the root. Again, it's normal to see this if the diseased gum is shrinking and getting healthier.

The small dark brown or green spots on the tooth or root are called calculus. Calculus both contributes to, and is formed as a result of, gum disease. Bacterial products and enzyme breakdown cause the inner gum lining to ulcerate. The lining bleeds, and the blood, together with plaque and dead cells, hardens and forms a deposit on the side of your tooth, like "scale" on the sides of ships. More bacteria live and cling to this calculus, so it's a good idea, after flossing and brushing correctly for several weeks, to visit your favorite dental office and get this hard, ugly material removed from your teeth.

Self-Testing

To determine if you have gum disease, here are some clinical tests that you can make, just as though you were a dentist. If you actually do what I next describe to you, rather than just read it, you may save yourself hundreds and possibly thousands of dollars over the years!

First, take the index finger of one hand and use it to help hold back the upper lip. Now, with the index finger of the other hand, press firmly on the upper gum with the tip of your other finger, and slowly move the pressing finger down toward the tooth over the gum triangle (papilla). See if it bleeds, or if you get a thin milky-whitish yellow fluid from the gum space. If so, this may be pus. After you've been plaque-controlling for a few weeks, this exudate, or fluid, should be diminished or gone. But you'll still need to have it

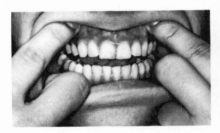
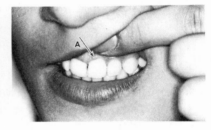

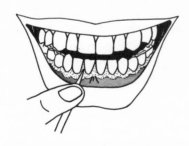

1. WHAT YOU SHOULD SEE IN THE MIRROR

2. TESTING WITH FINGER FOR GUM SPONGINESS

3. USE OF A BLUNT TOOTHPICK WILL INDICATE GUM SPONGINESS

4. 5. DENTAL FLOSS CLEANING WITHIN GUM SPACE

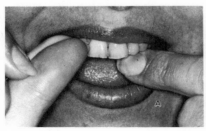
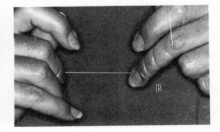

checked at the dental office with the probe to make sure that there isn't a pus pocket present.

The next test is to press on the gum gently with a dull toothpick (bite off the point). See if the gum has resistance to your pressure, or is very soft and spongy. If soft, it needs toughening up with plaque control and gum compression techniques, which I'll describe shortly. If it's shiny, it's probably soft. Healthy gum is textured with a stippled appearance, like an orange peel, and light doesn't reflect easily from its surface.

Next, take some dental floss and try to pass it into the gum space. Wrap the floss (a piece about fifteen to eighteen inches long) around the middle fingers of each hand. Now, using the index finger of each hand, place the floss between the lower two front teeth, and slide it alongside one of the teeth into the gum space. Allow it to go down into the gum space until it meets some resistance. Then slide back up and out. Smell it. Does it have a very bad odor? Now think of bad breath. That's where most bad breath comes from—The gum space. If you're not flossing regularly, you may really be knocking out your friends and family. In addition, you're letting bacterial-infection products enter your bloodstream. *In* fact, in a recently described report of patients suffering from fever of undiagnosed origin, it was found that the fever in many of the patients was due to localized infection in the gum. Once the infection was removed, with the aid of periodontal treatment, the fever was eliminated.

Having inserted the floss into your gum space, did the gum bleed when you removed the floss? Most people not flossing regularly would get some bleeding. Because most people get it doesn't mean it's normal. It's not. It indicates disease. Most people do have ulcerated gum linings. That's why the gum bleeds when you brush or floss. Fortunately, if it's a mild situation, it is reversible.

Keeping a Record: The Key to Long-Term Health

We have now completed our visual examination. How did you do? Let's write down in a table how you did now, and compare it with a once-a-week check for the next three weeks, after you start your plaque control. If you stop now, do your own examination, and take the time to write down what you see, you have taken the most important step to having a healthy mouth. By filling in this table, you are making a commitment to yourself to continue with your new knowledge.

At the beginning, your answers may all be "yes." After two weeks most should be "no."

	1ST EXAM DATE		1 WEEK LATER DATE		2 WEEKS LATER DATE		3 WEEKS LATER DATE	
	YES	NO	YES	NO	YES	NO	YES	NO
CONTOUR NORMAL								
GUMS SHINY, NOT STIPPLED (NO ORANGE-PEEL TEXTURE)								
GUM BLEEDS FROM FLOSS OR BRUSH								
GUM OVERGROWN BETWEEN TEETH								
GUM IS REDDISH AT MARGIN								
FLOSS PLACED UNDER GUM HAS STRONG SMELL								

PLAQUE CONTROL

Now that you've given yourself an examination and score for the first exam, let's get on with the business of getting those gums healthier. We do this with plaque control. Plaque consists of many bacteria living together in a meshwork of sugars, proteins, saliva, and other junk. It sits on the teeth, and especially likes to rest in the area just under where teeth touch, next to the gum margin, and within the gum space.

Remember, even though you can't see it, healthy gum has a small space between the tooth and the gum lining. The space is called a *sulcus*. It is similar to the space between a fingernail and the soft tissue of the finger. As disease progresses, the space gets deeper and fills up with more bacteria.

Staining

To help you see the bacterial plaque, I suggest you get Q-Tips, or make them by rolling small bits of cotton around a few toothpicks. Next, we need something called a *disclosing agent*. This is usually a dye that stains bacteria. Most frequently it's a red dye. Go to the drugstore and ask for disclosing solution or tablets. Butler Company's "Red-Cote" tablets or liquid is an example. If you find the red color inconvenient, you might try another product, Plak-Chek. With Plak-Chek, the dye is yellow and less visible until viewed under a blue light. I personally prefer a solution as it's less messy, but tablets will work. (If you're in a place with no disclosing solution or tablets, your pharmacist can make up a mixture for you. Ask him for a 1 percent gentian violet solution, or a tincture of iodine solution. Both will stain bacteria, but gentian violet is more dramatic.) If you're going to use the red disclosing solution, place your Q-Tip or cotton-tipped toothpick into just enough solution to saturate the cotton. To make disclosing solution from disclosing tablets, you can:

> 1. Make a solution of thirty disclosing wafers added to seven fluid ounces of warm distilled water and one fluid ounce of alcohol (95 percent).
> 2. Allow one half-hour for tablets to dissolve.

Now paint the edge of your gum where it meets the teeth and move the Q-Tip along, up and down, following the gum line. Now do the same for the opposite jaw. To help reach all your teeth without staining your lips and cheeks, use either the index finger of your other hand to pull your lip out of the way, or use the dental mouth-mirror that some drugstores sell. It's okay if you use disclosing tablets by chewing one up and swishing around. I find they get everything red, including your tongue, so I prefer disclosing solution. (See Directory for addresses from which to order products.)

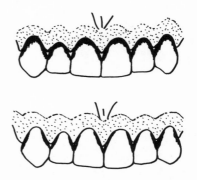

EVIDENCE OF STAIN AFTER APPLICATION

Now that you've stained your teeth at the gum edge with one of the systems described above, rinse your mouth with water and spit it out into the sink with running water. Now go to the mounted dental mirror (or Floxite lamp or Plak-Chek) and look to see where the stain is. It will most likely look like the illustration above. Now brush your teeth. Use any method you'd like. Now go back and look at your teeth again. If you followed the procedure correctly, you should see this: you'll notice that although brushing removed some stain at the direct edge of the gum, you did not get all of it between the teeth. (For those of you who think you did, you were fortunate to get out as much as you did, but there is still some left between the teeth where you can't see). For all of you, the reason you didn't get all the stain off is because the toothbrush doesn't reach all the way in between the teeth. Only dental floss will get into those areas to remove the bacteria. Brushing won't! That's why flossing is so important.

The most important point about staining—and it is the key to a healthy mouth—is to stain every third night, forever. By seeing the actual bacterial plaque, you'll be constantly reminded to remove it, and you'll remember to floss. The trick to keeping your mouth healthy is staining and flossing, not just brushing!

We've all been brainwashed to brush. It really hasn't worked well. Partly because of our poor diet. Partly because of incorrect brushing techniques. And . . . we were not taught to floss as children! Therefore, flossing is not automatic, or a habit, with adults. We need continued reinforcement. (Me, too!) I find by using the stain every third night, I can't fool myself.

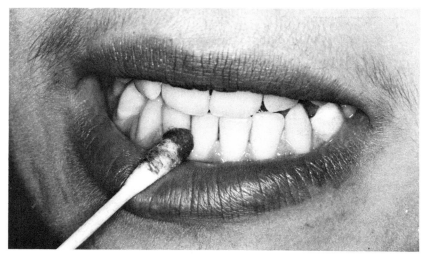

STAINING WITH A Q-TIP

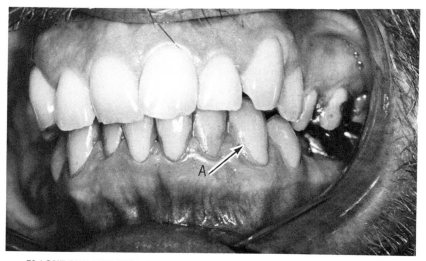

PLAQUE BUILDUP SHOWS UP AFTER BRUSHING, FLOSSING, AND STAINING

The Dental Prevention Kit

O.K. So you've stained, and now recognize the problem. What do we do about it? First, you get your dental kit together. It should consist of:

1. some waxed or unwaxed nylon, or silk, **dental floss**;

2. a **toothbrush** with three or four rows of .007 round, soft nylon bristles. Many companies market this kind of brush. You may want to try a few different styles to find the one most comfortable for you. Some have rubber tips on one end as an additional aid for massaging the gum between the teeth. A typical example is shown in the illustration below. Don't use natural bristles or medium or hard brushes for the brushing method I'm going to describe. (See Directory for product information.)

3. A round **toothpick**, or better yet, a **Stim-U-Dent** (purchased at the drug store).

4. Most important, is our **disclosing solution** or disclosing tablet. You'll need to use this to check your effectiveness every third night and later for spot reviews and reinforcement.

The other items, which we already have, are the dental mouth mirror and our viewing mirror. Let's look at all the items we're using: (1) mouth mirror; (2) viewing mirror with flashlight (or Floxite or Plak-Chek); (3) soft nylon brush; (4) dental floss; (5) staining solu-

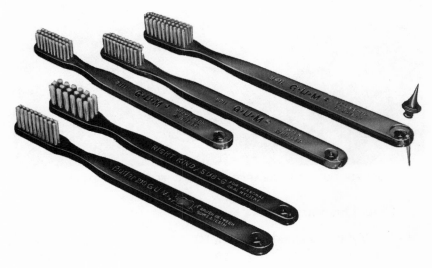

BUTLER GUM BRUSH

tion; (6) round toothpick or Stim-U-Dent. Now that you have all the ingredients for your Save Your Teeth Kits, you can get started.

Proper Gum Brushing and Tooth Brushing

To help you gain familiarity with the method for removing plaque, first start with the *brushing technique*. But for only one reason. You're used to toothbrushing, and you can see immediately, as you stain and then brush, how effectively you are removing the plaque. Interestingly, you're going to see immediate results. Bleeding should decrease, and your mouth will start to feel better, healthier, and cleaner. After brushing, I'd like you to stain again, and see if you've missed anything. If so, where? Then go back and try to remove it.

Using a soft, nylon bristle brush with rounded .007 bristles, place the brush at a forty-five degree angle, aiming the bristles down on the lower teeth or up on the upper. Just remember that as a memory aid when getting used to the new brush technique. Aim *up* for upper teeth, and *down* for lowers. The bristles actually enter the gum space. Now move the brush side to side a short distance—approximately one quarter inch, not more—in a "shimmy," or quick, light, scrubbing motion. It should look like the illustra-

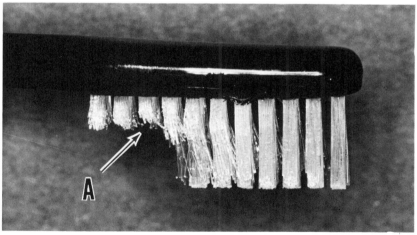

BRUSH WITH ROWS OF BRISTLES REMOVED TO ALLOW CLEANSING BEHIND LOWER FRONT TEETH

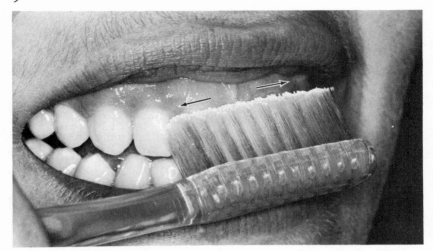

SOFT TOOTHBRUSH AT 45-DEGREE ANGLE MOVING ¼″ SIDE TO SIDE

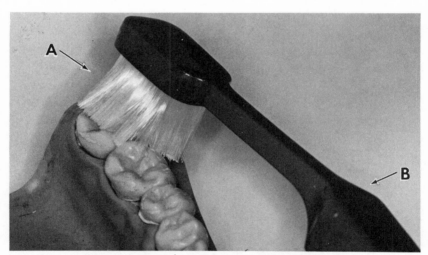

BRUSH POSITION, REAR TEETH, 45-DEGREE ANGLE

tion above. Do this for a count of eight. Then switch to the next group of teeth. It is most natural to begin in the upper left or upper right rear, on the cheek side, and work section by section until you have completely gone around the arch. Whichever side you start on, always try to do it from that side first, so you can develop a routine.

When you've finished the upper, turn your brush upside down and place the bristles in the forty-five degree angle-position, aiming down into the gum space next to your lower teeth. Again start to brush the gum-space section by section, for eight counts each. Generally, you'll find you will be able to cover about three teeth per series of short, horizontal brushings, so you'll probably shift areas about five or six times as you go completely around the arch.

One important suggestion: For gum brushing, don't use toothpaste. Since it's the mechanical action of the brush bristles that we want to clean in the gum space, more plaque is dislodged with a dry brush than one with a whole glob of toothpaste on it. Toothpaste is

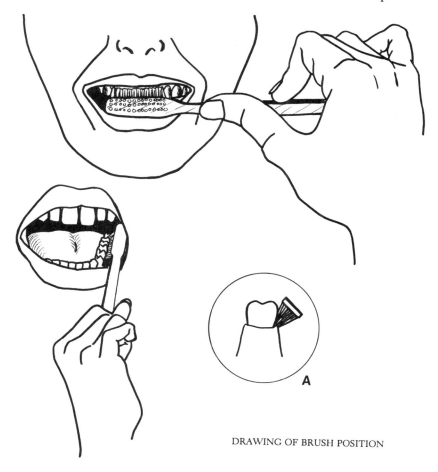

A

DRAWING OF BRUSH POSITION

important for other things, later, when you brush your teeth, you can put on the toothpaste.

When you've finished brushing the outside gum, open your mouth wide, place the brush, bristles turned up, on the inside surface of your upper teeth, where the gum from the palate meets the tooth. Hold the bristles fairly vertical, almost in the same direction that the tooth grows. When you feel *maximum penetration of the bristles in the gum space*, you've found the best angle for you. Now "shimmy" the brush horizontally for a count of eight; then change brush position six times as you go around the arch, the same as you did before. When finished with the upper, turn your brush bristles down, insert the bristles between gum and tooth, feeling for the best angle of maximum penetration, and start brushing. I recommend that for the inside lower teeth, the bristles be almost vertical with the tooth, rather than at the forty-five degree angle. It seems to allow for maximum penetration. For brushing the teeth themselves, either a side-to-side or up-and-down motion is O.K. The brush should be almost at a right angle to the tooth surface. For the tops of the teeth, a back-and-forth scrubbing motion is fine.

Well, now you have it. One extra suggestion: If your lower front teeth form a narrow arch and you can't get the entire brush head in, I suggest you get a second brush, cut off one-third of the bristles toward the handle, and with this smaller brush, you should have no trouble getting into the lower-front problem area. Johnson & Johnson has now come out with a smaller toothbrush for children called "Youth"! This can help reach difficult areas.

After you've finished brushing, stain your teeth and see how well you did. Try to see where you've missed, and try to get the remainder off.

How often should you brush? I would suggest twice a day, with the morning and evening being the most likely times. Technically, best results are obtained if you brush within twenty minutes after finishing a meal, because after that the bacteria are already too advanced in their production of plaque acids. You might keep a toothbrush at work to brush after lunch. The most important point is to remember to stain after the evening brushing, to test your plaque-removing ability.

You might want to try some of the newer brush designs that are

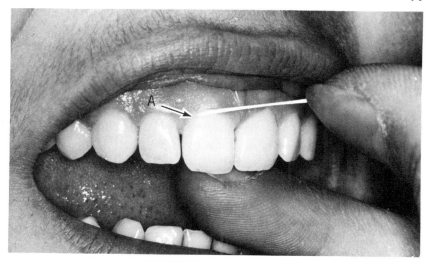

FLOSSING THE UPPER TEETH

now being manufactured. The design of the head has been made smaller in some to reach more difficult areas. In addition, several manufacturers have changed the angle of the bristle so that the bristles penetrate into the sulcus more easily. These two changes are particularly helpful for the molar teeth and the inside lower front teeth. An example of this type would be the "Reach" toothbrush shown below. This smaller head is particularly good for children or the small mouth of an adult.

Another excellent product for cleaning between the teeth of your bridge is the Proxabrush by Butler. It is a spiral-shaped brush that helps remove plaque between teeth, like a toothbrush. Butler and others also make a useful device to hold floss as you insert it between the teeth, if you have difficulty with your fingers. Two of the better-known products of this type are Butler's Floss-Mate, and Floss-Aid.

Flossing

Don't start flossing until you're sure you've got staining and brushing down well. When they're easy for you, go on to flossing.

By the way, when flossing first was heavily emphasized, unwaxed floss was recommended. Since then, comparison studies of waxed versus unwaxed floss have found no definite difference. So I would suggest that as long as the floss is strong and thin, either should be O.K. for you. I personally use unwaxed because the floss splays, creating many fine fibers, as you move it up and down. I seem to find it does a better job in my mouth.

The method of holding the floss is as follows:

1. Unwind a string of floss about eighteen inches long.
2. Loop one end around the middle finger of one hand, and the other end around the middle finger of the other.
3. Keep gathering up the floss on both fingers by rotating your middle fingers in a circle toward each other, until they are about three inches apart.
4. For the upper arch, most people use both thumbs, or the thumb and index finger, to hold the floss. Place one thumb (or index finger) just behind the teeth (inside your mouth) and the other thumb outside. The closer the fingers are held, the more control you'll have over the floss.

To do the upper teeth, the floss is gently inserted between the teeth with a back-and-forth motion until it passes beyond the tooth contact. It is then slid up along the tooth surface until it enters the gum space as far as it comfortably can go. The floss is moved up and down a short distance with gentle firmness against the side of that tooth. Sometimes you can hear a "squeaky" noise when this is done well. After three up-and-down passes, the floss is gently carried down and across the gum papilla, and into the adjacent gum space. You next clean the adjacent tooth with three up-and-down passes. You then slide the floss back and forth as your fingers move downward, so as to remove the floss from between those two teeth. Now the floss is passed between the next two teeth. The procedure is repeated until all tooth-to-tooth surfaces have been cleansed. Even

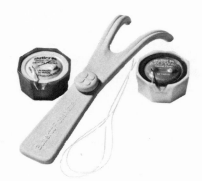

BUTLER BRUSH-MATE

if a tooth is sitting alone, its rear side and front side should be flossed into the gum space. Once you have mastered the technique, get into the habit of starting from the same tooth. I suggest starting behind the last tooth on the upper right and working around to the last tooth on the upper left.

Do not be alarmed if you notice bleeding from the gum lining when the floss goes in. Most people have this. It means that the gum lining is ulcerated. The bleeding should stop after several days of flossing. It is harmless, and each time you floss, as you bleed a little for the first few times, you are reducing the inflammation. It's sort of like letting excess air out of an overfilled tire. When enough excess air is out, the tire rides better. Same with the gum. You'll see in a few days that it's pinker and firmer, and that the bleeding has stopped.

When you've finished the upper arch, take another piece of floss, eighteen inches long, and prepare to do the lower arch. Instead of your thumbs, I suggest using your index fingers to help slip the floss between the teeth. Otherwise, the technique is the same. Using the index fingers as a guide, again slip the floss into the gum space and move the floss firmly up and down one side of the tooth facing the gum papilla, and then the other tooth surface facing the first one.

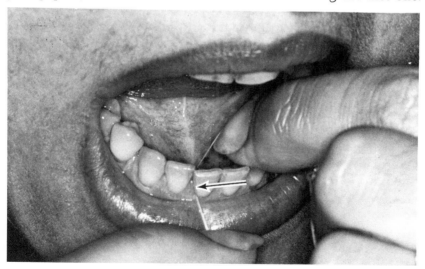

FLOSSING THE LOWER TEETH

I know this is not easy to learn, and if, after trying several times, you feel you're not getting the hang of it, call your local dental society or dental school. Ask them to help you locate a preventively oriented dental office near you where you can go for plaque-control training, if your present dentist is not involved in teaching plaque control, or if you have no dentist.

Practice

Remember, practice makes perfect. Flossing is a skill that requires patience and dexterity. Some people can do a very effective job of flossing their entire mouth in four minutes. Others may take twenty. It's not the time, but the final result that counts—so stain your teeth after flossing and see how you did. Whatever time it takes you to floss, I guarantee that as you do it daily, you will get faster and faster. If you stick to it, flossing may ultimately take you only four minutes for each dental arch. You might make it easier for yourself by doing it while watching television. This way, it's not taking extra time, and can be fit more easily into your life-style.

After several weeks of flossing just once a day, you should find that any puffiness or bleeding of the gums has subsided, and your breath should be much fresher. For those of you with fixed bridges who can't floss through tooth-to-tooth contacts, the Butler Company makes a product called the EEZ-Thru-Floss Threader, which seems to work very well. It is used by inserting the dental floss through the round loop, again using a piece of floss about eighteen inches long. The little plastic tail of the floss threader is inserted under the solid contact between the two capped teeth that are connected. The tail is passed from the cheek side toward the tongue side, caught by the thumb and index finger of the other hand, and then drawn out of the mouth for about six inches. You now have the floss between the teeth,

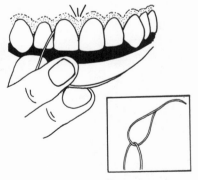

USING THE BUTLER EZ-THRU FLOSS THREADER

and can floss into each gum space as described earlier. When finished with flossing, simply pull through and out of your mouth. The threader is used wherever teeth are connected, and where the floss can't be passed directly between the teeth.

OTHER GUM AIDS AND HOW TO USE THEM

What about other aids to gum health? Two excellent aids are the interdental wood stimulators or "compressors." One is called a Perio-Aid, and the other, Stim-U-Dent. Here's how each works.

The Perio-Aid

The Perio-Aid is a plastic handle with two ends, each with a hole to receive a round toothpick. A green collar screws tightly onto the toothpick to secure it. The toothpick should extend only about one half inch out from the handle. If you can't get a Perio-Aid, ask your drugstore to order some for your community from the Marquis Co. (See Directory.)

Directions: Insert a round toothpick through either hole of the Perio-Aid from the side that has numbers (1 or 2). Insert the toothpick through the hole from the number side, until one half inches sticks out the other side. Tighten the green collar against the toothpick, and pull the long part of the toothpick down against the green to break it off. The Perio-Aid is now ready for use. It will look like the illustration on page 60. For upper teeth, the handle is best held vertically, for lower teeth, horizontally. The toothpick should be inserted through the #2 hole for the outside gum, and the #1 hole for the gum facing the tongue inside the mouth. The toothpick point is used by inserting it horizontally between the teeth and compressing the gum. Push up on the upper gum, and down on the lower gum. The compression helps toughen the gum and reduces inflammation. The toothpick point can also be used as an aid to cleaning in the gum space. Some dentists feel it is good for removing plaque. I personally feel that it may remove some. However, it is so large in comparison to the size of the bacteria that it plays less of a plaque-removal role than does flossing and brushing. On the other hand, the

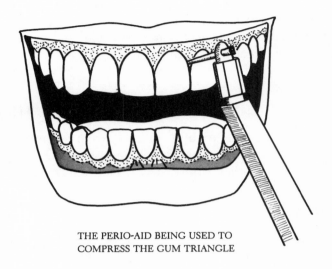

THE PERIO-AID BEING USED TO
COMPRESS THE GUM TRIANGLE

Perio-Aid toothpick, or a hard rubber interdental stimulator, similarly shaped, does wonders for compressing the gum, helping reduce
inflammation. I have found that the Perio-Aid seems to have an advantage in results over "rubber-tipping." I feel the entire benefit in
firming up the gum is a result of the better compression from the
harder wood. The gum seems to respond more quickly, and after
using the Perio-Aid for a while, the gum stays closer to the bone.
The Perio-Aid should be used on both the outer gum and the inner
gum.

Stim-U-Dent

Another product that firms the gum is the Stim-U-Dent. Its one
disadvantage is that it can only be used for the outer gum (on the
cheek side). It is excellent for compression, convenient (you can easily carry it in pocket or purse) and is easy to use. For those who can't
get a Perio-Aid or don't want to, go to your pharmacy and get a
package of Stim-U-Dents. They are a must for helping shrink your
inflamed gum. They are held between the thumb and index finger,
while balancing the other three fingers on your chin. About one
inch of the Stim-U-Dent should emerge between the thumb and

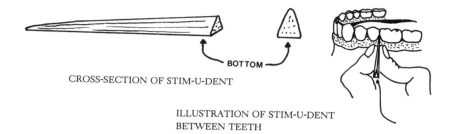

CROSS-SECTION OF STIM-U-DENT

BOTTOM

ILLUSTRATION OF STIM-U-DENT
BETWEEN TEETH

index finger aimed toward your teeth. The bottom of the Stim-U-Dent faces down for the lower teeth, and up for the upper. The bottom is recognizable because it is less wide in cross-section than the other two sides of the Stim-U-Dent. The motion in using the Stim-U-Dent is to insert it inward between the teeth until you feel compression on the gum. Do this three times, in-out, in-out, in-out, until you feel pressure each time. Then move to the adjacent tooth, and start again. You'll get faster with practice and the results are worth your effort.

As with flossing, the Perio-Aid and Stim-U-Dent, when first used, can cause gum recession if the gum is inflamed. This will stop in a few days, especially if done in conjunction with proper flossing and brushing. It's a big help for rapid results, so use one or the other.

One other word of advice: If your gum triangles (papillas) fully occupy the space between your teeth, don't force the wood tip in too hard. Just apply light pressure to the tip of the gum. Don't wedge it so firmly that you'll ultimately create a space, except as naturally occurs from inflamed gum shrinking. You'll find that if you have crowded teeth where brushing and flossing are not reaching well, the Perio-Aid will help.

Water Irrigators

There are basically two types of irrigators. One is attached to the faucet and is powered by the flow from the tap. The other is a self-contained unit driven by a motor-operated pump that supplies water in a pulsating jet. Each manufacturer claims superiority. They are both useful, but at a lower level of effectiveness than flossing or brushing, for the following reason. Neither really removes plaque. They both help dislodge food debris and loosened plaque, and may also dilute harmful products at the surface layer of the plaque. But they don't remove it. They are particularly helpful for people with extensive dental work in their mouths—such as lots of crowns and bridges—or children with braces. The Water Pik is one such pump-operated irrigator that has been found effective. A faucet type, called Assist-Dent, is made by Clairol.

POINTS TO REMEMBER

That's it, then. Flossing, brushing, staining, the Perio-Aid, Stim-U-Dents, and water irrigators all have been described. Keep using the chart for weekly recordings of your progress, and keep staining.

You're going to be amazed at the rapid results. Don't forget my suggestions regarding your dental examination, including probing. Dental X rays do not show enough. Until your dentist has probed, you really won't know whether you need further definitive gum treatment. So, after working on your own mouth for three to four weeks, make that appointment for a thorough periodontal examination with your dentist or a periodontist. We'll discuss what a thorough examination consists of later on. For now, let's see how we can have healthy teeth.

THREE

How You Can Have Strong, Healthy Teeth

HAVING HEALTHY TEETH as an adult necessitates having started off with good dental habits and good food as a child. Most of us did not, because certain information wasn't available when we were kids. This chapter will discuss

- how we got where we are
- what we can do to help prevent our children from having as much breakdown as we had
- how as adults we can eliminate further breakdown

SEQUENCE OF ERUPTION

Let's review for a moment what I said earlier about decay. You can't have decay until you have teeth, and that requirement is met somewhere between the ages of six and fourteen months, when incisors (front teeth) erupt. Usually the bottom front teeth erupt first, then the top front come in, and other teeth later erupt until there are a total of twenty teeth, ten in each jaw. Eruption is usually complete by the age of three years. Missing or extra teeth are not uncommon, and can lead to *malocclusions*. A malocclusion is the incorrect meeting of the teeth of the upper and lower jaw. So count your child's teeth and, if in doubt, check with your dentist.

FACTORS INFLUENCING WHETHER DECAY OCCURS, AND AT WHAT RATE

Once the teeth have erupted, there are several factors that will influence whether decay occurs, and at what rate:

Tooth Eruption Dates

PRIMARY TEETH

NAME	AGE AT ERUPTION	AGE AT LOSS OF TOOTH
Upper		
Central incisors	8–12 mos. 10 mos. (±2 mos.)	6–7 yrs.
Lateral incisors	9–13 mos. 11 mos.	7–8 yrs.
Cuspids (canines)	16–22 mos. 19 mos. (±3 mos.)	10–12 yrs.
First molars	13–19 mos. 16 mos. (±3 mos.)	9–11 yrs.
Second molars	25–33 mos. 29 mos. (±4 mos.)	10–12 yrs.
Lower		
Central incisors	6–10 mos. 8 mos. (±2 mos.)	6–7 yrs.
Lateral incisors	10–16 mos. 13 mos. (±3 mos.)	7–8 yrs.
Cuspids (canines)	17–23 mos. 20 mos. (±3 mos.)	9–12 yrs.
First molars	14–18 mos. 16 mos. (±2 mos.)	9–11 yrs.
Second molars	23–31 mos. 27 mos. (±4 mos.)	10–12 yrs.

PERMANENT TEETH

NAME	AGE AT ERUPTION	ROOT FORMATION APPROXIMATELY COMPLETE
Upper		
Central incisors	7–8 yrs.	10–11 yrs.
Lateral incisors	8–9 yrs.	11–12 yrs.
Cuspids (canines)	11–12 yrs.	14–15 yrs.
First bicuspids (premolars)	10–11 yrs.	12–13 yrs.
Second bicuspids (premolars)	10–12 yrs.	13–14 yrs.
First molars	6–7 yrs.	10–11 yrs.
Second molars	12–13 yrs.	15–16 yrs.
Third molars (wisdom teeth)	17–21+ yrs.	approximately 20 yrs.
Lower		
Central incisors	6–7 yrs.	9–10 yrs.
Lateral incisors	7–8 yrs.	10–11 yrs.
Cuspids (canines)	9–10 yrs.	14–15 yrs.
First bicuspids (premolars)	10–12 yrs.	12–13 yrs.
Second bicuspids (premolars)	11–12 yrs.	13–14 yrs.
First molars	6–7 yrs.	10–11 yrs.
Second molars	11–13 yrs.	14–15 yrs.
Third molars (wisdom teeth)	17–21+ yrs.	approximately 20 yrs.

1. The mother's diet during pregnancy, as well as her state of health during pregnancy.
2. a. The presence or absence of fluoride in the drinking water as the child's teeth are forming and calcifying. The child must drink fluoridated water as part of his/her diet, or the parent must add fluoride to the diet with vitamins, or add drops with measured fluoride content to water, juice, or milk. This will allow fluoride to reach the tooth while it is mineralizing and help the enamel form a harder, more decay-resistant crystal.
  b. Application of topical fluoride—applied by the dentist with twice-yearly cleanings using stannous fluoride paste, followed by topical application of stannous fluoride solution or acidulated phosphate-fluoride solution or gel.
  c. Topical fluoride applied at home, via toothpaste, mouthwash, or fluoride gels in trays for home use.
3. Oral hygiene—you do it for your baby and for your child, until he/she is old enough to take over; and do it yourself.
4. Diet: The baby's diet, the child's diet, your own diet, particularly eliminating sugar. The baby's diet is best coordinated with a pediatrician. No baby bottles should be left in the mouth for any extended period of time. This is especially true for nighttime sleeping.

As you can see, several of the above considerations were not available to you when your own teeth were forming. Possibly you had a bottle in your mouth for too long as a baby, so you got off to a worse start than your kids.

THE MOTHER'S DIET

The pregnant mother should be eating well during her pregnancy to ensure healthy development of the fetus. We will discuss diet and nutrition in the next chapter. Basically, it consists of eating balanced meals and having some food each day from each of the four basic food groups (dairy; fruits and vegetables; meat, fish, or fowl; and cereal—whole-grain breads).

In addition, I recommend a good, well-balanced multivitamin, multimineral preparation as a supplement.

Among the things you should not take by mouth, or systemically, is tetracycline. If, as a pregnant mother, you happen to get sick, and your physician wants to give you an antibiotic, don't take tetracycline. It can stain the baby's first set of teeth. Similarly, don't let the child be given tetracycline up to age twelve, as that can stain the primary and permanent teeth while they are developing. When they come into the mouth, they may be yellow instead of white.

Since the first trimester of pregnancy is the one during which developmental defects in the fetus are most likely to occur, it is best not to drink alcohol or take drugs or medication during this period particularly. It generally would be best not to take any of the above, but to help avoid having a deformed child, at least eliminate these items during pregnancy, especially the first three months.

SYSTEMIC FLUORIDE

The question of whether or not fluoride passes the placental barrier, getting to the baby from the mother's bloodstream, is currently being reevaluated. New evidence indicates that fluoride may pass through the placental barrier. If so, it might be important that the mother-to-be drink fluoridated water daily. At present, it is still felt that the major benefit of fluoridated water on the developing teeth occurs after the baby is born.

Under optimum conditions, a tooth comes into the mouth with 800 ppm (parts per million) of fluoride in the outer layer of enamel. Though good, that level does not get the tooth surface to its hardest state, which would be 1,000 ppm in the outer surface. Therefore, in addition to using fluoridated water, it helps to add fluoride topically to the baby's and child's teeth, as they grow. Even as adults, there is a constant interchange between the surface of the tooth and the saliva, and using a fluoride toothpaste helps maintain surface hardness and resistance to decay.

It's very important to know if your water supply is fluoridated, and how many ppm of fluoride are present if it is. Ideal is 1.0 ppm. Acceptable is .7 to 1.3 ppm. Your pediatrician, dentist or pedodontist should be able to answer this question. If he doesn't know, ask him to check with the local board of health's dental division. It will influence whether or not you administer additional fluoride via drops in water or juice, or in the form of vitamins. This extra fluoride should only be added to the water the baby drinks if the water supply doesn't have fluoride, or if the level is too low. It should also only be done under the supervision of your dentist or pediatrician. This is to make sure that the baby doesn't get too high a dose of fluoride, which could lead to a funny-looking discoloration of the teeth called *mottling*. For this reason, if you use a formula for a child, check to see if fluoride has been added, and if so, how much. If your water is fluoridated and the formula is fluoridated, you may go too high.

FLUORIDE APPLIED TO TEETH SURFACES

Since it is known that enamel is most resistant to decay when it has more fluoride incorporated in its surface layer, we should know the best methods of applying fluoride to the teeth for surface penetration. Please note that in all liquid applications to the teeth, it is essential that the teeth first be cleaned of plaque. We want the fluoride to go right onto the enamel and it would defeat our purpose if the teeth were dirty with plaque. O.K., let's see what can be added to clean the teeth surface and introduce fluoride. The first item works for everybody, both kids and adults. It's. . . .

Toothpaste

This is the most obvious cleaning method and, at the same time, the most common method of hardening the outer tooth surface. As a topical application, it is also the least effective for fluoride intake, although it does help. What toothpaste should be used? Any fluoride toothpaste bearing the seal of approval of the American Dental Association Council on Dental Therapeutics is fine. Crest has particularly been recommended. I feel that research I've seen on Aim is also rather convincing, and makes that toothpaste a good vehicle for the fluoride. There are others. For example, Colgate with MFP is very effective. The key point here is to help your child brush the plaque away. First use a dry brush, which is more effective mechanically. Then, when you think that the teeth are clean, use the fluoride toothpaste.

Fluoride Mouth Wash

When the child is old enough, and can handle swishing and spitting out easily, a fluoride mouthwash can be used. You can get this from your pharmacist or dentist. It has been shown to be effective in reducing decay when used as directed, by rinsing or, in certain cases, swallowing. Caution here! Only permit swallowing if there is no fluoride in the water and if your dentist has prescribed the mouthwash, and be sure of the allowable dosage. Again, brush the teeth clean first. For younger children, after cleaning the teeth with dry gauze, bathe them with a gauze or cotton ball impregnated with the fluoride solution.

Visits to the Dentist

The third leg in the multiple attack on decay is a semiannual visit to the dentist from age two years on. He can clean the teeth with a stannous fluoride-containing paste, and then apply a special solution to harden the enamel even more. One such solution frequently used is stannous fluoride. Another is an acidulated phosphate/fluoride solution or gel. These are each applied after the teeth have been thoroughly cleaned. The period of application is usually four minutes. The child is told not to eat, drink, or rinse his mouth for thirty minutes following treatment. It is advisable to have this type of treatment once every six months, from age two to fifteen, for maximum benefit to all teeth.

Oral Hygiene

Proper oral hygiene must be started early. Bacterial plaque is present on the tongue and on the gum pads of the baby. It should be removed once a day even before the teeth erupt. The procedure may be started after a few months, using a piece of gauze or the corner of a washcloth. After the last feeding, simply wipe the gum pads. When the teeth erupt, it will be into a cleaner area. Continue to do this during and after eruption. When the child is about two years old, a soft nylon baby-size toothbrush may be substituted for the gauze. Until the age of six or even seven, you should brush and floss your child's teeth, as he lacks adequate manual dexterity. The best way to position yourself is to stand behind your child or put his head on your lap. Use the soft toothbrush and brush his teeth the same way you brush yours. Once a day, use dental floss from the same position. As he gets older, you can introduce disclosing solution. Let him brush first, then point out where he missed. He might brush with toothpaste; then you allow him to disclose, and see where he missed. Go over those areas without toothpaste. Before letting him do it on his own, make sure he has mastered both brushing and later flossing. Make sure he knows how to use disclosing tablets and/or solution, and that he does it twice a week. You might provide an incentive by telling him that on occasion you will spot-check him with disclosing solution. If he has no stain (and therefore no plaque), he wins one dollar. This gives him a goal, and he will save you plenty of dollars by reducing his dental bills.

It has been estimated that by using communal water fluoridation, removing plaque from your child's teeth, having the dentist or pedodontist clean the teeth with a stannous fluoride paste twice a year, (followed by use of stannous fluoride solution or acidulated phosphate solution or gel for four minutes), and regular home use of a toothpaste such as Crest, Aim, or Colgate MFP, the incidence of dental decay can be cut by at least 75 percent in both children and adults.

DIET

Eliminate sugar

It's one thing to make the tooth as hard as possible, but even the hardest tooth will dissolve if we bathe it in enough acid. But don't take my word for it. Put the next tooth you can get hold of (one of your children's that has come out; or maybe you could ask your dentist for a tooth that he has removed) in a glass of soda and check it out in two or three days. You'll find it soft and rubbery. If soda can do that, think of what all the sugar foods are doing to that poor tooth surface. Every time you eat candy, sugar, honey, refined flour products, dried fruits, sweetened cereals, ice cream, canned or frozen fruit in syrup, hard candy, puddings, sodas, etc., you're just bathing your teeth in acids. The acids come from the bacterial plaque working on the sugar.

There's another factor to consider. It's not only the amount of sugar or refined carbohydrates you take in, but also the frequency. If, in addition to the three meals you have normally, you also nibble or have snacks, then those also can contribute to your decay. Coffee and doughnuts, which many people have for breakfast or a mid-morning snack, are killers. Ice cream cones, which are delicious, and probably the most universal American snack food, are also very unhealthy because of their sugar content. J. Yudkin, in his book *Sweet and Dangerous*, has given strong evidence that sugar is more involved in causing heart disease than cholesterol. Yet the figures on national consumption of sugar today are staggering. The average American today consumes over 120 pounds of sugar a year. In Chapter 1, I have listed the foods commonly eaten and their sugar content. Please study that table again to see what you're doing to yourself!

So now we've covered the basic areas that you can influence to produce sound, hard, undecayed teeth. They are:

1. Community water fluoridation
2. Good prenatal diet for mother
3. Topical fluoride or other tooth-surface hardeners:
   a. Toothpaste
   b. Mouthwash with fluoride once a day
   c. Six-month cleaning with stannous fluoride paste and topical application of fluoride at same visit (from age two to age fifteen)
4. Good diet for the baby, coordinated with your pediatrician
5. Reducing sugar in the diet, especially sticky forms of sugar
6. Changing types of snacks to sugarless snacks—fruits, veg-

etables, or nuts instead of candy, ice cream, potato chips, and soda (see Chapter 4).

CHALLENGING SOME DENTAL MYTHS

What other questions might be raised about the teeth themselves? Let's examine some of the frequently asked questions, and explode some myths.

1. Does pregnancy ruin teeth? Does it take mother's calcium to build up the baby's bone and teeth?

Absolutely not. Your bones would give up the calcium before your teeth ever demineralized. And your diet and metabolism would have to be extraordinarily disturbed for that to happen.

2. Why do teeth sometimes appear worse after a pregnancy?

Usually because the mother isn't taking care of her mouth. She's not brushing enough, not aiming carefully, and not flossing. Many pregnant women notice that their gums tend to bleed in the eighth or ninth months, some earlier than that. Again, this is because plaque is not being removed, and the bacteria are irritating and breaking down the gum. During the first three months, a pregnant woman may have cleanings and simple dental procedures. It is important for the pregnant woman to continue her own minor dental care during her second trimester of pregnancy. Extensive dental work can be deferred until after the baby is born, but decay should be eliminated, and tartar removed, if present, during the fourth through the sixth month.

3. Are some people born with soft teeth?

No. On rare occasions, there are developmental, or genetic, peculiarities in the formation of the enamel, or dentine. But these are not common. The usual comment about soft teeth refers to a child, or to an adult who, when younger, kept getting cavities, went to the dentist, kept getting cavities, and so on. If carefully checked, these people would be found to have had poor diets, lots of sweets, poor hygiene, frequent snacks of foods containing sugar, little fluoride protection, and so on. Their teeth weren't soft when they came in, but they got soft because of poor habits and lack of preventive measures.

4. What else could contribute to tooth breakdown or deformation?

Fevers of the mother or drugs taken during pregnancy, or in the first year of life of the newborn, can affect the shape of the developing tooth buds and the mineralization of crowns. The pregnant mother is advised to have as pure a diet as possible. I would eliminate stimulants such as coffee, tea (unless herbal), smoking, drugs, medications, food additives, and stress.

It is not easy when a child is born and something is wrong to go back and figure out what did it. Worse still, it doesn't solve the present problem. So it's best to keep the odds in your favor when pregnant by eating carefully, getting lots of rest, avoiding undue stress, and getting lots of easy exercise—walking, swimming, bicycling, and so on.

5. You keep stressing the harmful effects of sugar. But it tastes so good, and kids just seem to find ways to get candy. How can I control this?

The best way—set the example. Eliminate sugar from the house, and if you must use a sweet substitute, use the tiniest amount of honey possible. Try to use minimum amounts of sugar substitutes.

Don't bribe kids with sweets as a reward for good behavior.

If you want to give them candy or ice cream, make it on Sunday, at a definite time, so they know that's the only time it's acceptable. Like two or two-fifteen P.M. If they don't develop the taste for sweets, it'll be much easier not to overindulge and wreck their teeth.

6. If you get a toothache just once, and it goes away, is it all right to ignore that tooth?

No. It is very dangerous to ignore a toothache, even if the pain goes away quickly, because teeth have to be pretty broken down before you'll even feel something. Appreciate the toothache as a warning signal to run to the dentist and let him check the tooth to see what caused it. It's the best way to prevent big trouble, and save the tooth.

7. What is "nursing bottle syndrome"? Why is it destructive to a baby's teeth?

Children with this problem usually have very badly decayed upper front teeth. The decay can be bad enough to have spread to the back teeth, and so extensive on each tooth that parts of the tooth have just melted away. The problem arises because the baby is allowed to take the bottle to bed. Usually the bottle has milk, juice, or perhaps jello water in it. When the child falls asleep sucking, the liquid forms pools around the upper front teeth. The mouth is warm, the bacteria are there, and there is a decreased flow of saliva during sleep. The bacteria form acids from the liquid food, which cause the teeth to rot. The decay can be so bad that the teeth are rotted to the gum level. In the earlier stages, the teeth can be saved by the dentist. Later on, they may be causing infection and abscesses and may have to be removed.

You can help prevent this by nursing the baby while he or she sits up. Try to eliminate the bottle altogether, or place water in the bottle at night. Tongue-thrusting, which leads to separation of the front teeth, can also develop from staying on the bottle too long.

Lastly, bring your child in for a dental examination at approximately eighteen months, rather than at three years.

8. If my child's teeth come in late, is he (she) going to be a slow learner?

No. In fact, teething may be easier, and you can also help by keeping the mouth clean with gauze pads while the teeth erupt, to lessen the discomfort. But there is no relationship between delayed tooth eruption and intelligence.

9. Is it okay to pull a decayed baby-tooth if it's rotten and hurting?

Try to save it first. Ask the dentist if it could be filled, or have root-canal work done and have it capped. If the tooth can be saved, the child is better off because the primary teeth (baby teeth) serve as guides for the eruption of the permanent teeth. If the tooth is missing, other teeth may shift, or tip, and block out the permanent tooth. Or the permanent tooth may come in, but in the wrong position. So try to save baby teeth, especially the back ones, whenever possible. If it has to be removed, be sure to ask about space maintainers (see Chapter 9, in the section on pedodontics).

10. Which primary teeth don't need space maintainers and which do?

The front teeth, if lost, don't have to be replaced for dental reasons. This is because there will be no loss of space in the front of the mouth.

The rear teeth, if lost, have to be replaced by a space maintainer because they guide in the six-year molar. If not replaced, tipping and shifting take place. If that happens, the permanent adult tooth coming in may be blocked out or may come up in the wrong position. The first permanent molar, which comes in at age six, has been called the key to the occlusion. Primary molars must be kept until ages eleven to twelve to keep the six-year molars in the correct position.

HOW YOU CAN HAVE HEALTHY TEETH AS AN ADULT

Now that we've discussed your child's teeth, you can see where your own mouth might have been led astray. Of course, you'd like to know what can be done for your teeth now.

1. Eliminate sugar and refined carbohydrates. Sticky foods and sugar-containing foods cause decay.
2. Reduce the number of snacks. If you do snack, eat fruit, vegetables, salad, nuts, seeds; or drink water. All are healthy and won't cause decay.
3. Plaque control. Brush twice a day, after meals (especially after breakfast and dinner. Make sure that you floss daily. Stain every third day to see how you're doing. Keep score at the beginning.
4. Use a fluoride toothpaste recommended by the American Dental Association.
5. If any roots are sensitive, rinse daily with a fluoride mouthwash and brush with Sensodyne toothpaste.
6. Have your dentist check your teeth for cavities, either new ones or under old fillings. If you're getting lots of cavities under old fillings, and your diet and plaque control is good, think of switching dentists. Well-filled teeth should not keep decaying. It means either that you aren't doing your job with mouth cleanliness and diet, or your dentist isn't doing his.
7. *Make sure your teeth are probed periodontally every six months.*

Either your dentist or periodontist can do this. Make sure he *records the numbers as part of your record,* so he can compare the numbers with previous and future visits. If things aren't written down, the memory deceives. Ask him whether any numbers are over "3," and if so, what he plans to do to help reduce the gum "pocket" to a normal reading. These numbers are important. They are measurements in millimeters of the gum space in health or disease. Generally, there are three clinical criteria for periodontal disease. The first is bleeding from the gum lining when the probe is placed. The second is the depth in millimeters that the probe goes before the dentist or periodontist reaches the bottom of the gum space. Readings of 0–3 mm are generally considered normal; 4 mm means that there has been some gum breakdown that has usually not yet involved the bone; 5–8 mm means that the bone is involved, but the tooth can be saved; 9 mm frequently means that the future of the tooth is questionable; and 10 or higher usually means extraction of the tooth. Thus you can see that these readings are very important diagnostically to determine the extent of gum treatment. The third clinical test is the presence of exudate, as described in Chapter 2. If you or your dentist, by pressing a finger against the gum, can "milk" a whitish-yellow fluid from the gum space, then that gum area is probably diseased.

FOUR

The Right Diet for Strong Teeth and Bone

IF YOU ARE like most people, you would like to feel healthy and full of energy all of the time. You would like to sleep well, and feel that you could easily play several sets of tennis, or run a few miles, or swim for an hour at a time. But can you? If your life depended on having to run two miles without having a heart attack, could you do it? If you're like most people, the answer is no. The reasons for this have to do with two areas: nutrition and physical fitness. Your body and your mind ultimately reflect what you do for them, and if you eat poorly, it's like throwing a mixture of gas and water in your car's engine. The car may run, but not very well.

The same is true of internal glandular fitness, organ fitness, and muscle fitness. If you don't work your body continually, gradually, and systematically, you're not pumping it with enough blood to cleanse the wastes it produces. Nor are you using your body enough for it to maintain a state of readiness and fine conditioning. Thus, when a physical stress or emergency comes, your body may disappoint you.

What does all this have to do with teeth? Plenty. The health of the teeth, particularly the gums and bone, depends a great deal on proper diet and proper nutrition. Your ability to repair any damage caused by bacterial products or aging is a function of your nutrition, absorption, utilization, circulation, and your general resistance. Thus your cellular health is greatly influenced by your diet. Your diet is everything you eat, while nutrition means which foods you eat, how much, their composition, your body's needs for nutrients, and how they are used as your body assimilates the vitamins, minerals, and foods in your diet.

NUTRIENTS

To understand what nutrition is all about, let's first consider the word "nutrients." Nutrients are chemicals in foods, which provide you with energy, and build and maintain your tissues, organs, and various parts of your body. Nutrients are also necessary to help regulate the functions performed by all parts of your body.

Scientists have classified nutrients into six types: carbohydrates, proteins, fats, minerals, vitamins, and water. Each type of nutrient, except for water, includes many individual nutrients or life-sustaining substances. If all of these nutrients are not present in adequate amounts, your body's ability to produce energy efficiently or to repair tissue may be greatly reduced. Let's see how you can have a healthy mouth in a healthy body by planning and maintaining a proper diet that includes these essential nutrients.

DESIGNING YOUR DIET

Understanding proper dietary information will allow you to design a diet that is both enjoyable and healthy. Poor food selection can be instrumental, along with other factors, in contributing to such diseases as tooth decay, gum disease, heart disease, diabetes, hypertension, and poor resistance to infectious diseases.

You'd probably like to know what foods, and how much of these foods, you should eat to be well nourished. Actually, this depends on many factors, including your age, height, weight, sex, physiologic state (Are you pregnant? Or perhaps highly athletic? Or very sedentary?), and your genetic inheritance.

YOUR REQUIRED DAILY ALLOWANCE (RDA)

The Food and Nutrition Board of the National Research Council has established the Recommended Dietary Allowances (RDA) for six minerals, ten vitamins, proteins, and calories, as revised in 1974. These RDAs are set at levels which supposedly will assure good nutrition for most normal people. Although they may assure good nutrition, there is some question as to whether they will provide optimum nutrition.

THE FOUR FOOD GROUPS

Some years ago, to make dietary recommendations that would help the public eat more nourishingly, a guide was developed called "The Four Food Groups." It was adopted by the Department of Agriculture in 1958. It classifies foods into the following four groups:

>1. *Milk Group:* Two or more glasses or equivalent daily, depending on age and physical state (e.g., pregnant or lactating).
>2. *Meat Group:* Two or more servings daily.
>3. *Vegetable and Fruit Group:* Four or more servings daily.
>4. *Bread and Cereal Group:* Four servings daily are suggested.

The idea with this guide is that if you eat foods daily from each of the groups as suggested, you should be getting a well-balanced diet. Here are representative foods from each group.

The Milk Group

This group includes such items as milk, buttermilk, skim milk, cheeses (including skim milk cheeses), butter, and yogurt. Milk fortified with vitamin D probably has more nutritional value than any other food, except perhaps raw eggs. It provides calcium, phosphorus, protein, vitamin A, and B-complex vitamins. Milk is a very poor source of iron, and many women are iron-deficient. Therefore, some iron supplementation may be necessary. Unfortunately, there are two additional qualifications for you to consider in drinking milk. The first factor is lactose intolerance. One third of the American people are lactose intolerant. Lactose is the natural sugar found in milk. If you are lactose intolerant, your symptoms may include gas, nausea, headaches or diarrhea, cramps, and excess mucus formation. Fortunately for those with this problem, a new product has been devised that eliminates the intolerance. It comes under various names, e.g., Lactozyme, Lact-Aid etc., and should be available in your nearest health-food store.

The second factor to consider regarding milk intake is whether your milk product is high in saturated fat. Although small amounts of fats are necessary in the diet to produce sex hormones and bile, and to help absorb calcium and carry vitamins A, D, E, and K into the bloodstream, too much fat is dangerous as it may lead to obesity, clogged arteries, and heart disease. Nutritionists generally agree that it is best to consume low-fat dairy products, particularly low-fat fortified milk. Cottage cheese is an excellent low-fat dairy product, since it is rich in protein and has most of the saturated fat removed.

The Meat Group

The meat group includes lean muscle and organ meat, fish and other seafood, poultry, eggs, beans, peas, seeds, nuts, or nut butters.

This group provides protein, iron, niacin, and other vitamins and minerals. The basic building block of protein is the amino acid. For a diet to be well balanced, all the "essential" amino acids should be included and be in the proper proportions. Proteins from certain sources, for example, dried beans, peas, and nut butters, are not biologically "complete." Consequently, if you get more protein from vegetable sources than animal sources, your diet should be balanced so that the meal has all the nutrients needed. For example, adding milk or a milk product to a meal of vegetables would greatly increase the protein value of the meal. A meal of brown rice and beans is a good source of protein, and the two foods combined contain almost all essential amino acids. On the other hand, meat, fish, poultry, and eggs have all the desired "essential" amino acids.

It would be a mistake to conclude that it's fine to eat as much meat as you want, as studies in the past few years indicate that if too much meat is eaten, one may ingest too much saturated fat. While it is true that meat is very high in protein one can obtain the necessary amount of protein from other sources. Fish, turkey, and chicken without the skin provide good protein without too much fat. One may also get protein from nonflesh sources such as eggs, dairy products, seeds, and nuts. In fact, many groups of people in the world, for economic or religious reasons, never eat meat. Studies of several groups who eat little or no meat (i.e., the Hunza and Ecuadorians) have shown that meat is not necessary for a balanced diet, assuming that the combination of proteins from nonmeat sources provides the full complement of essential amino acids. Many nonmeat-eating, agrarian people show extremely good health, which most likely also relates to their being very active physically. Pritikin's research at the Longevity Institute in California seems to bear this out. He recommends a diet high in complex carbohydrates, low in animal proteins, and extremely low in fat.

The Vegetable-Fruit Group

This group includes all fruits and vegetables. It is from this group that we get both our vitamins and minerals in great quantities, as well as some fiber for bulk in the stool and some protein. If possible, vegetables and fruits should be eaten raw; if cooked, steaming vegetables with very little water is the best way, as this preserves most of the important vitamins and minerals. For those of you who are interested in eating healthy vegetables and have a "green thumb," I suggest that you get into "sprouting." See the Bibliography for a suggested text. Sprouts are fun to grow and are very healthy to eat.

Vegetables usually are divided into the green leafy and deep yellow groups, and are rich in vitamins A, B, and C. Potatoes, with the skin, are among the most nourishing "starch" vegetables. Since most people do not eat enough vegetables and fruit (and that includes those of you who eat only lettuce-and-tomato salads), it is necessary to stress one key point. Four or more servings daily from the vegetable-and-fruit group are recommended for good health. If you just have an evening lettuce-and-tomato salad and think that you are getting enough B vitamins and vitamin C from that, think again. Remember this: the B vitamins and vitamin C are water-soluble and can't be stored in the body. Therefore, you are only able to use that which you ate that day.

Here are some excellent sources of the water-soluble B and C vitamins:

> 1. *B vitamins:* Liver, wheat germ, yeast, bran, brown rice, whey, and soybeans. Many other foods contain varying amounts of the different B vitamins, but the above foods contain almost all of the B-complex vitamins in the necessary amounts.
>
> 2. *Vitamin C:* Vitamin C is found in all citrus fruits. Some other sources of this vitamin are carrots, watermelon, celery, peppers, peas, tomatoes, apples, spinach, turnip greens, and collards.

The best sources of vitamin A (which is a fat-soluble vitamin) are liver, eggs, whole milk, fortified skim milk, fortified butter, and margarine.* Some other good sources of vitamin A in both the vegetable and fruit subgroups are apricots, papayas, peaches, mangoes, broccoli, Brussels sprouts, carrots, chicory, lettuce, beet tops, collard greens, dandelion greens, endive, kale, romaine lettuce, raw onions, parsley, red peppers, sweet potatoes, spinach, winter squash, tomatoes, turnip greens, and watercress.

The Bread and Cereal Group

This group includes breads, cereals, grains, pastas, and rice.

These foods provide a substantial amount of carbohydrates, a relatively inexpensive source of energy. Breads and cereals are also important sources of iron, B-complex vitamins, and some protein. Unfortunately, the majority of our packaged breads and cereals have been so highly milled that much of the iron and B-complex vitamins have been lost in the process. Thus, anything made with white flour, even though it is "enriched" (a term meaning that some lost nutrients have been replaced), is not as preferable for a nutritious diet as breads made from whole-grain wheat, oat, corn, rye, soybean, or rice flours. Brown rice and whole-grain cereals, especially those which

---

* Harold Rosenberg, *The Doctor's Book of Vitamin Therapy,* 1974, G. P. Putnam's Sons.

contain bran, a rich source of food fiber, are highly nutritious foods also.

Many people suffer from constipation, and in the past few years we have realized that our low-bulk diets have been largely responsible. Some bulk is obtained from fruits and vegetables, but much of the bulk here is from cellulose. Human beings, unlike cows, can't break cellulose down. Though cellulose helps clean the intestine, it can also be a little rough on it if we have too much. Bran works differently. It has the interesting quality of absorbing fluid, and as a result, it helps speed food transit time in the intestine and bowel and provides bulk, thus maintaining a good diameter in the intestine. The length of time it takes you to digest and to eliminate food you've eaten has been linked to cancer. If it takes you *more than* twenty-four to thirty-six hours, you're retaining fecal material which, when broken down, may produce some undesirable, potentially cancer-causing byproducts. Also, water is continually absorbed from the overretained stool, and it becomes dehydrated and hard. High-fiber foods will be helpful in maintaining real regularity. It's suggested that four servings daily from the bread-cereal group would give you your best dietary balance.

In addition to eating nutritiously, and getting enough vitamins and essential food materials, you might also be interested in your weight. Calories do count, so let's define a calorie.

CALORIES, PROTEINS, FATS, CARBOHYDRATES

Calories

Calories are a unit of measure that represents the amount of potential energy that foods contain and the amount of energy human beings (and other living things) require for growth and health. The source of calories in our food are *proteins, carbohydrates,* and *fats.* Pure proteins and carbohydrates of equal weight supply equal amounts of calories; however, the same quantity of fat contains over twice as many calories.

If you were to continuously consume an excessive amount of foods that supplied calories without any or relatively few nutrients that are essential for health, this could affect your dental health as well as the health of other parts of the body. These foods are often made from highly refined grains, frequently in combination with some sweetener. If the sweetener is retained on the surface of the teeth, mouth bacteria can convert the "sweet" into acid, leading to decay.

Your age, sex activity, current weight, and degree of physical activity help determine the proper number of calories you should consume in your diet. The best way to judge if someone is getting the correct number of calories is by growth for children and appropriate weight and change of weight for adults.

What do you need to be healthy and repair well? You need good-quality proteins, fats, complex carbohydrates, minerals, and vitamins. Let's examine each for a moment.

Protein and the Essential Amino Acids

Proteins are the basic building blocks of tissue. They form connective tissue and muscle, and are in almost all parts of our bodies, including bones. Protein is also required for proper functioning of our bodies and is one of our sources of energy.

There are many different proteins in foods. These proteins contain different combinations and amounts of some of the various amino acids. Human beings can synthesize some of these amino acids, while other amino acids must be present in the foods we eat. The most complete foods contain all the essential amino acids in the proper proportions; others either have only some of these essential amino acids or not enough of them. The complete foods are milk, cheese, fish, poultry, meat, and eggs. As already stated, vegetable proteins are not complete and require balancing with additional nutrients supplying the missing essential amino acids. For example, milk or cheese could supply the missing ingredients.

Fats

Another key nutrient is fat. Fats are a group that fits into a larger classification called *lipids.* Lipids are classified as triglycerides, phospholipids, derived fats, and sterols. We don't recognize familiar foods in this classification, yet each of these represents something we know well, such as cholesterol.

Let's make some basic points regarding fat and your diet:

1. The American public consumes too much fat, and even a government subcommittee has introduced a recommendation that as a nation, we reduce our fat intake from 40 percent of our diet to 30 percent.

2. Excess fat intake has been linked to obesity and heart disease.

3. Certain diets have recommended losing weight by eating as much protein and fat as one wanted, as long as carbohydrates are eliminated. This should be done only under the care of a physician and only for a short time period.

4. Margarine, once thought to be safer than butter, has now been shown to have had such changes made to it in preparation, such as hydrogenation, that it is considered more likely to be cancer producing than ordinary butter. Ordinary butter was originally reduced in the diet beause of concern regarding heart disease.

5. Cholesterol, which has been linked to heart disease, is produced by your own intestines and liver. The consensus among several authors concerned with heart disease is that dietary cholesterol should be restricted, but not totally eliminated. As mentioned above, if your diet was cholesterol-free, you would still have some in your bloodstream because your liver and intestine produces it.* Cholesterol is needed to form bile salts and the steroid adrenal and sex hormones. In the skin it serves as a precursor of vitamin D. It also facilitates the absorption of fatty acids from the intestines.†

In summation, current recommendations regarding fat are that "with care, some low-cholesterol or low-fat diets can be beneficial if they are also low calorie. The secret is to have a low-calorie, high-nutrition diet."‡

My specific recommendations regarding fats in your diet are:

1. Reduce the amount of fatty foods and increase the amounts of

---

* Robert C. Atkins, *Dr. Atkins' Super Energy Diet* (New York: Crown Publishers, 1977).
† Benjamin T. Burton, *Human Nutrition* (New York: McGraw-Hill, 1976).
‡ Richard A. Passwater, *Supernutrition for Healthy Hearts* (New York: The Dial Press, 1977).

fish, fowl, vegetables, fruit, whole grains, and cereals consumed in your diet.

2. Eat a small amount of unsaturated fatty acids daily. One teaspoon of safflower oil used on salad or vegetables daily is a beneficial source of these fatty acids. In addition, some authorities recommend thinning the saturated fats unavoidably absorbed into the bloodstream by sprinkling a tablespoon of granulated lecithin on your cereal, or taking it with yogurt and some fruit. The lecithin is thought to aid in the transfer of the blood fats in a soluble form, so that they do not tend to deposit on blood-vessel walls.

3. Exercise more. Get into this by slowly increasing your daily amount of exercise. An excellent book to help you get in shape is Morehouse's *Total Fitness in 30 Minutes a Week.* *

4. If you're overweight, reduce both carbohydrate and fat intake. The "weight watchers' " diet is a reasonable diet and may be used as a general formula upon which you can improve.

Carbohydrates

In less developed countries, complex carbohydrates constitute a much greater source of calories than in highly industrialized nations. If you eat complex (in other words, nutrient-rich) carbohydrates, then as long as you have some high-quality protein, your diet should still be adequate. It is the relationship between calories taken in and calories burned up that determines whether you stay at the same weight or keep gaining. Some of the longest-lived people have high-carbohydrate diets, with heavy emphasis on grains and dairy products. They are frequently very physically active and this activity continues well into old age.

In the more developed countries like the United States, we have a major problem because the percentage of *refined* carbohydrates is much too high. Of the refined carbohydrates (cake, candy, ice cream, white bread, cookies, etc.), those foods containing sugar (sucrose) are the most dangerous. Sucrose is totally devoid of vitamins

* Laurence E. Morehouse, *Total Fitness in 30 Minutes a Week* (New York: Simon and Schuster, 1975).

and minerals. It has been shown to be responsible for most tooth decay, plaque development, and nourishment of bacteria. It has been related to the increase in heart disease, to diabetes, and to obesity. Carbohydrates supply energy, but the best ones for a balanced diet are those that are in foods that also contain minerals, vitamins, and some protein (in other words, complex carbohydrates such as whole grains or whole potatoes). By combining high-protein foods with a small amount of unsaturated fats and nutrient-rich carbohydrates in our daily diets, it is possible to achieve an increase in your energy level while maintaining good health.

VITAMIN AND MINERAL SUPPLEMENTS

Without vitamins and minerals, you could not function. Many important biochemical reactions can only be completed when vitamins and minerals assist in the transfer of atoms and molecules as we metabolize. Vitamins are classified as either water soluble (the Bs and C) or fat soluble (A, D, E, and K). Water-soluble vitamins can't be stored in the body while the fat soluble ones can. If you don't eat enough whole-grain vegetables and fruits, and drink enough fresh water, you are not going to get enough of the minerals the body needs to function properly. You have heard of iron-deficiency anemia as one common mineral deficiency. Liver, organ meats, egg yolks, and meat generally will help supply iron (which is a particularly important mineral for adult women, who need more of it than adult males). Of all the nutrients, this is the most frequently deficient.

Vitamin deficiency occurs when our diets are deficient in the essential vitamins needed for good health. Because American diets have been inundated with refined foods, hidden sugars, processed foods, food preservatives, and food additives, some diets may be inadequate in certain vitamins or minerals. Most nutritionists feel that if people eat the RDA (Required Daily Allowance) of vitamins and minerals, they will be adequately nourished. Others feel that this is a generalization that may not be adequate for a given individual whose metabolism may require higher dosages than usual.

There has been great controversy in the past few years regarding vitamin and mineral supplements. After reading numerous books on the subject, my conclusions are:

1. The Required Daily Allowance (RDA) should come from foods, with vitamin and mineral supplements used only *as* a supplement, not as the primary source for nourishment. Although the RDA for vitamins is possibly adequate to sustain life, it may not be sufficient to allow you to function at maximum efficiency, with maximum energy, and with maximum ability to repair. I recommend *Super Nutrition* by Richard A. Passwater as probably one of the best books you could read to help you determine your true needs and what supplement dosages of vitamins and minerals are right for you.*

2. Although many scientists still argue as to whether vitamin C does or doesn't stop colds, the work of Linus Pauling and Irwin Stone indicates to me that supplemental dosages of vitamin C, balanced throughout the day, are probably best for most of us. I recommend a basic 2,000 mg per day taking 500 mg. in four doses, one with each meal and one before bedtime.

3. Vitamin and mineral supplements should be taken with meals. Since the vitamins and minerals act as linking factors, helping reactions between chemicals to occur, they work best when they are taken with or just after one's meal. Then they can combine with the food products as they are broken down and digested.

4. There should be a proper ratio of calcium to phosphorus in the body. But most people eat and drink so many foods containing phosphorus that they frequently have too little calcium (many "sodas" are phosphate-rich and calcium-poor). Since calcium is needed for good teeth, strong bones, and muscle contraction, a deficiency can produce many problems. An adult should be getting 800 to 1,000 mg per day.† If you're not, drink more milk, eat more cheese, or add some calcium supplement.

5. Overdoing vitamins: Are there any dangers in taking too much? Yes, although the upper limits are much higher than previously thought. The RDA recommended dosage for vitamin A, for exam-

* Richard A. Passwater, *Supernutrition for Healthy Hearts* (New York: Pocket Books, 1976).
† Benjamin T. Burton, in his *Human Nutrition* (New York: McGraw-Hill, 1976), recommends 800 mg. Atkins recommends 1000 mg. U.S. RDA is 1000–1500 g per day. (Ref.: *Federal Register*, Volume 38, No. 148, Aug. 2, 1973.)

ple, is 5,000 units for men and 4,000 units for women. Many people routinely take 40,000 to 50,000 units with no side effects. On the other hand, there have been reported deaths or severe illness from taking above 100,000 units for long periods of time. Since vitamin A is stored in the liver, it is probably not advisable to take more than 25,000 units daily on a continuing basis. This 25,000 units includes food intake also. Vitamin D should not be taken in excess either. This could happen when foods fortified with vitamin D are eaten in addition to medicinal vitamin-D preparations or excess vitamin intake. So you should not exceed 400 units per day totally.* The water-soluble B and C vitamins really can't be overingested in that they are eliminated by the kidney and liver when taken in excess. Naturally, if you consume too many supplements over a long period of time, the possibility does exist of damaging the kidney or liver by overtaxing their excretory ability. But this would have to be in extremely high megadoses. There have been reports that large doses of vitamin C can destroy vitamin B_{12} under laboratory conditions. This has not been confirmed in human studies. There have also been reports that large intakes of vitamin C may lead to dependency on large maintenance dosages. Others deny this. To put it mildly, the vitamin C controversy is still very much alive.

What processes destroy vitamins? Excess cooking destroys vitamins. Smoking cigarettes has been shown to reduce the vitamin-C level in blood tissue, and stress causes a much greater utilization of the B and C vitamins. Infections also place greater demand on the body and rapidly use up the vitamin pool. Birth control pills disturb the metabolism of many vitamins and minerals, and should probably not be taken without vitamin and mineral supplements.

DIET AND TEETH

Now that we've discussed nutrition and some generally useful information, let's focus specifically on the mouth. There are several basic concepts to consider:

* Ken Keyes, *Loving Your Body*, 1966, New York, Frederick Fell, Inc.

1. Nutrition of the pregnant female.
2. Baby's nutrition after birth.
3. Which foods cause cavities and why.
4. What can be done to reduce cavities caused by poor diet.
5. How does the diet affect periodontal health?

It's a sad comment that there are approximately 110,000 dentists in the United States primarily involved in treating dental breakdown, that over $6 billion a year is spent on mouth care, and yet we are still losing the battle. Here's how to help yourself:

1. If you are pregnant, remember that the food you eat is also being used to nourish your fetus. From the second month to the end of pregnancy, an extra 30 g of protein per day is recommended. A lactating (nursing) mother must have at least 1,200 mg of calcium daily, because she may lose up to 300 mg in her milk. She should be sure during pregnancy and nursing to eat amply from the four food groups so as to obtain a balanced diet. I would also recommend a good, balanced multivitamin, multimineral preparation to insure adequate nutrition.

2. After birth, a major opportunity to get the baby started off with healthy teeth and bones begins. Fluoride, which did not pass the placental barrier, should now be given to the baby either via the community water supply, vitamins, or drops in the formula. Ideally, one aims for the baby to have 1 ppm of fluoride daily. This should be done with the help of the pediatrician and family dentist, as discussed in Chapter 3. Also, look at the baby's actual diet and see where the food itself could produce decay. We know that sucrose (sugar) is Public Enemy No. 1 when it comes to causing decay. Try to eliminate sugar. Here are some other major points:

1. Sticky solid foods with sugar are worse than liquids with sugar. (For example, candy bars are worse than cola drinks, but both are bad.)
2. Sugar taken with a meal does not seem to increase the number of cavities as much as sugar taken between meals. Therefore, carbohydrate snacks will tend to increase the

amount of decay, and if the snack consists of sugar in a sticky form, the decay will be even worse.

3. Different foods produce decay at different rates. It is the kind of food, when it is eaten, and with what other foods it is eaten, that ultimately determine its contribution to decay.

From the above, it is obvious that to control a high decay rate, you should immediately:

1. Lower or eliminate intake of sugar.

2. Reduce the number of highly refined carbohydrate or sugary snacks. Make sure that the snack has as little food in it as possible that is sticky or adhesive. Raw fruits, vegetables, and nuts are excellent snacks.

3. Satisfy the need to have "something sweet" as a snack, by having it for dessert right after your meal. If you have a high decay rate, after the meal, brush with a fluoride toothpaste, floss, and then rinse with a mouthwash containing sodium fluoride designed for rinsing.

4. Stain the teeth daily. Make sure all plaque is removed.

5. Visit the dentist and have him remove all decayed areas and restore teeth with fillings and dental restoration as needed.

6. Twice a year, have a cleaning with fluoride paste at the dental office, followed by topical fluoride application.

7. Have any virgin teeth treated by odontoplasty (a simple modification by your dentist of the biting surface of rear teeth to eliminate grooves that trap bacteria).

8. The use of sealants will also help to reduce decay in pits and fissures.

What about the supporting structures of the teeth—the gum, the bone, the periodontal ligament? How do nutrition and diet influence the health of these tissues? The periodontal tissues are in a constant state of flux and are composed of living cells and intercellular material. They are nourished by the blood supply. They are subject to damage in two ways: direct and indirect.

Direct damage can occur if the diet contains foods that stick or adhere to the tooth next to the gum. Bacterial plaque then forms more rapidly, and this in turn causes gingivitis (gum inflammation). Bacterial plaque is also fed by secretions from the lining wall of the gum. If this is diseased, then breakdown products from the gum lining as well as blood leaking from the gum lining both serve to nourish the bacteria. Several studies have shown that the bacterial composition in the plaque can be changed for the better just by altering your diet. In addition, since your resistance to gingival breakdown, as well as your ability to repair, is directly influenced by the digested food products and vitamins brought to these areas, it follows that the better nourished you are, the better able you are to resist breakdown. Where the periodontium does start to break down, it will be able to repair more rapidly. There is some feeling among nutritionists that older people may be calcium deficient. Intake of more milk products or calcium supplements would help remineralize the tooth-supporting bone to some degree if one is calcium deficient. However, without removing bacterial plaque and pockets, all the calcium supplements in the world won't stop periodontal disease.

In summary, we can say the following: The nutrition of the pregnant mother influences the structural formation of the baby's mouth tissues as well as the teeth. The baby's diet influences the mineralization of the teeth, and their tendency to decay or not decay. This is particularly influenced by how many sugar-rich snacks the baby and/or child has between meals and what mealtime foods are eaten. All dietary influences can be modified positively by good plaque control (brushing, flossing, and staining), as well as fluoride application (toothpaste, rinses, and dental visits for topical fluoride application) to harden the tooth surface.

The gum health is indirectly influenced by how much decay has occurred in the past, because no filling is ever as gentle to the gum tissue as your own tooth. All restorations collect more plaque than the tooth itself, and plaque causes gingivitis. Secondly, the diet may contribute directly to plaque formation leading to gingivitis. Lastly, your diet will influence your resistance to cellular breakdown and your ability to repair the results of breakdown. If I may use an old cliché, "You are what you eat."

I sincerely believe that nutrition is not a complicated area for you to study, and that if you do undertake to eat properly, the rewards are great. As the Chinese have said, "A journey of a thousand miles begins with a single step," so start your journey by rereading this chapter a few times, read the references cited, and keep on reading. You'll continually grow and be feeling better all the time. The journey may take a lifetime, but it'll be a longer, healthier lifetime.

FIVE

How You Can Get from Birth to Dentures Without Really Trying!

BIRTH DEFECTS

Putting together everything we've discussed so far, we now can see that there are several factors that influence how the mouth breaks down. The first few months of pregnancy are the months when major organs are forming and tissues differentiating. If the mother's diet or health suffered, major birth defects in the mouth could occur. This could lead to harelip or cleft palate, salivary gland abnormalities, malformations of the shape of the jaws and the joints, and later, deformities in the shapes of the developing teeth. These deformities can be caused or influenced by materials entering the mother's bloodstream and passing the placental barrier to reach the developing fetus.

For this reason, before eating or drinking something, the pregnant woman should really ask herself: "Is it a natural substance? Could it affect the developing baby?" Among potentially dangerous and commonly used materials, one would include smoking, medications such as aspirin, sleeping pills, any mild or strong narcotics, liquor, tranquilizers, barbituates, and so on.

THE YOUNG BABY

Fluorides

Once the baby is born, depending on the amount of fluoride intake, the child will have hard, mineralized teeth to a greater or lesser degree. We discussed the "baby bottle syndrome" as a major cause of rampant decay in the upper front teeth. This decay is a result of leaving the child with the bottle when he or she sleeps. If the bottle contains milk or juice, and it collects around the teeth, the bacteria will create acids within twenty minutes, and this will start to decay the teeth. It is best to give the baby a bottle with plain water if you feel that it still has a need to suck, and let the baby nurse on the bottle as long as necessary.

Gum Pads

We said it is a good idea to wipe the gum pads in the front of the baby's mouth even before the teeth come in. This will keep the mouth clean and reduce pain from teething. Even after the teeth erupt, wiping the pads with gauze twice a day, after morning and evening feedings, will help reduce decay.

Thumbsucking

Once the front teeth are in the mouth and the swallowing pattern has begun to change (some time between twelve and eighteen months), one should try to remove the bottle and let the baby drink from a cup. This will help reduce the tendency toward thumbsucking.

Thumbsucking may be a result of generalized anxiety, or a habit developed during early nursing, or perpetuated from an earlier period, during fetal development. According to Moss,* children who suck their thumbs already had the habit well under way by the seventh month in the uterus. Thus the unborn baby is already exhibiting sucking and chewing movements, in preparation for nursing, even before it is born.

Sucking is a normal reflex for a baby. A child should be allowed and encouraged to work the tongue and cheek muscles as much as possible to achieve good muscular balance. This will help the teeth erupt into the mouth in good position. Thumbs and fingers are nature's pacifiers; they are around a long time. The disadvantage of a

* Stephen J. Moss, *Your Child's Teeth* (Boston: Houghton Mifflin Co., 1977).

manufactured pacifier is that it can be lost. The less the child uses either pacifier, the more likely the jaws and teeth will develop in good alignment. I suggest you read Moss's book regarding breaking bad habits, and speak with your own dentist or pedodontist if you are having difficulty. Breaking habits isn't easy, and requires a lot of positive reinforcement, as well as substitution of another pleasurable activity for the negative habit.

It would be best if the child had lost the habit at about age two and a half. The longer the habit persists, the greater the damage.

Some mothers wonder whether breast feeding or bottle feeding is better. If the mother's psyche is positively disposed toward breast feeding, it is definitely an advantage to the child. Human milk is a superior food to cow's milk (for humans). The child exercises his sucking muscles (tongue, cheek, lips, chewing muscles) more thoroughly, and lastly the child is held upright, the normal position for digesting, rather than on his back, as is frequently the case with bottle feeding. It's pretty tough to digest lying on your back. Try it!

The First Dental Visit

At approximately eighteen months, it would be a good idea to let the dentist clean the baby's teeth with a fluoride toothpaste, and begin topical application of fluoride to harden the teeth in the mouth.

Sugar

Let's avoid sugar. The less sugar, the better the teeth are going to be. Let's try to not get the growing child into the soda-pop habit. Let's try not to introduce candy or lollipops, hard sugar, or even soft or sticky sugar products because they taste good or shut the child up. The price you pay later is not worth that moment of relief from the child's nagging.

EARLY CHILDHOOD

Since the development of the child is greatly influenced by what he or she eats, try to feed the child by using the principles of the four basic food groups. Any good pediatrician who understands nutrition should be able to help you. Supplementing the diet with a good multivitamin or multimineral can only help, as very few diets are perfect even with the best of intentions.

Throughout the childhood years, the two key areas we are concerned with are (1) preventing decay and (2) allowing the permanent teeth to come into the mouth in correct position.

As the child grows, and decay occurs, early repair of the tooth to prevent its loss is important. If somehow a posterior primary tooth is lost, then the dentist or pedodontist should replace it with a space maintainer to help give the necessary room for the permanent teeth to erupt in place.

You would like to see your child with a healthy smile, with comfortable chewing, and with the proper dental relationship of each tooth to the next, and of the upper teeth to the lower teeth. You do not want to see crowded teeth, decayed or missing teeth, or dental problems like "buck teeth."

An early visit to the orthodontist, at about age 8, should help determine whether or not the permanent teeth are going to have enough room to come in straight. If not, then arrangements can be made to assist the growth and development of the permanent teeth into their correct positions in the mouth. This will help avoid costly and longer orthodontic treatment at a later date. It will also aid in the development of the form and shape of the face, jaws, and smile. If one starts orthodontics too late, like age thirteen years as used to be the custom, one can still change the bite; but no longer can you improve on the shape of the face.

Besides thumb- and finger-sucking, you should also observe whether your child is nail-biting, cheek-biting, lip-biting or tongue-thrusting. You may need professional help to break the habit, but once you recognize it, the earlier it's eliminated the better. The bones of the face can form in a certain position due to abnormal pressures from bad habits. Once they've formed, you can't undo the damage. *In tongue-thrusting,* for example, the child thrusts his tongue forward and pushes it against either his upper teeth, his upper and lower teeth, or the lowers only. The result is an opening between upper and lower teeth even when he closes his jaws to chew. This disturbs the protective function of the front teeth, puts extra pressure on the rear teeth, and is a major predisposing factor to a worse case of periodontal disease than would usually occur in the adult. Tongue-thrusting habits may be corrected either with the use of certain orthodontic appliances, or with myofunctional therapy. Abnormal swallowing habits are frequently outgrown. If your dentist, pedodontist, or orthodontist thinks that your child should see a myofunctional therapist, it would be wise to follow their suggestion. Some dental offices specialize in myofunctional therapy; many times it will be a speech therapist who helps correct abnormal speech, swallowing, or breathing patterns.

Tooth brushing introduction can begin as early as age two, but remember, it's an introduction. As the parent, you should still brush the child's teeth until he/she is five years of age. At that time, he/she can assume more responsibility. To make sure he is doing it, keep staining, maybe as frequently as every other day. You can help by seeing that your child develops the staining habit, and also by seeing how well he's doing in removing plaque. He'll learn by being involved.

TEENAGE DENTAL DESTRUCTION

So now you have a child with little or no decay, and with good teeth coming into his mouth in good position. If he needed orthodontics, you've helped him undertake treatment. So far his mouth is healthy? Can it still break down? Yes! How? Two ways: teenage eating habits, and teenage self-destructiveness and preoccupations with peer approval.

Many people think that they just have bad luck with their teeth. Their teeth are weak or soft. That's a myth. You have now learned what the proper building blocks to good teeth are, and obviously, if some or all the positive steps previously discussed are omitted, then the teeth are more likely to decay, or be crowded, crooked, or unsightly.

But even if your child gets to the age of twelve or thirteen in good dental condition, he or she now enters a very potentially dangerous age period for teeth. And if your child needs, or currently is undergoing, orthodontic treatment, then everything I'm going to tell you is doubly important.

At about age eleven or twelve, some very important and obvious changes are occurring in your child. I refer, of course, to puberty. Since I am not writing about puberty but about teeth, I want to alert you to a very important, but not obvious, change. It is at this age, eleven or twelve, that gingivitis seems to really take hold in most children. By age 13, 80 percent of the children in the United States have gingivitis. This means that 80 percent of the kids have inflamed gums. If this is not reversed, then most of these children or teenagers will get to their twenties and start losing bone. And in most cases there are no symptoms. Their gums bleed a little when they brush. It doesn't happen all the time. It goes away. There's no pain. And they're so preoccupied with more important struggles . . . for admiration and approval from their friends, wanting to be attractive to the opposite sex, doing well in school, and in sports. How can they even think about something that doesn't even bother them?

You can help them. If you've taught them how to stain for plaque, you've got them started on a very important habit. If you've taught them, or teach them, plaque control, good brush technique, and good floss technique, you're going to save them lots of time, anxiety, and possibly pain, later on in the dental office. And you're going to save yourself lots of money.

They get a second major benefit from staining and plaque control at this time. As puberty arrives, teenagers are growing rapidly and have large appetites. They eat lots of snacks. Frequently these snacks include junk foods. Keeping them focused on mouth care via plaque control will make it easier for you to explain to them that if they are going to snack, it's really important that they:

1. reduce or eliminate the number of foods containing sugar and refined carbohydrates;

2. substitute fruits, vegetables, salad, or hamburgers for candy and ice cream;

3. have sweets at home, rather than away from home, with meals, or as dessert, so it won't harm their teeth so much.

4. If they eat sweets at home, at least they can go into the bathroom and brush and floss after eating. If they get rid of the sugar within twenty minutes of eating it, it won't feed the bacteria, and thus the teeth won't dissolve.

Keep the teenager going to the dentist twice a year for cavity checks, cleaning with fluoride toothpaste plus topical fluoride application, and make sure he or she uses a fluoride toothpaste or similarly effective one.

But remember—any reversal of the good habits can start the breakdown again. Think of your mouth. Are you still requiring dental treatment? Do you still get cavities? Have you noticed that your gums are red, inflamed, bleed when you brush, or are receding? Has your dentist told you to come in more frequently so he can give you "gum treatments" consisting of scraping away tartar, and digging underneath your gums, making them bleed. *"Gum treatments" and scraping tartar away do not get to the cause of the problem. Those methods treat the results of the breakdown, the symptoms not the cause! They only help for a few days at best.* Cavities and gum disease can happen to you or your teenager if either of you stop daily plaque control, eat incorrectly, stop staining, and stop going to the dentist because nothing bothers you.

THE TWENTIES—A CRITICAL DECADE

I think of the years from twenty to thirty as critical years. They are the years of entrance into the work world, or into college and perhaps graduate school. They are years of intense preoccupation with major life-decisions regarding careers, possibly marriage, and the desire frequently to make it big in something—conquer the world, become rich and famous, or establish oneself.

Since one's mouth is usually not troublesome at that age, the young adult just tends to give it routine, superficial care. Here's what happens frequently.

His home-care brushing is superficial. He doesn't floss. He smokes. He eats poorly. He's under stress. Sometimes, at exam time, students break out in certain areas of their gums with puffiness, soreness, or easy tenderness, and stop brushing altogether because it hurts. This outbreak, sometimes called "trench mouth," (because soldiers used to get it during World War I in the trenches) is a result of two bacteria overgrowing and destroying tissue, especially between the teeth. If the gum breakdown is not immediately reversed on the first attack, then even after healing, the gum is left scarred. The area of greatest tissue destruction between the teeth may never regrow completely, and as a result a deep crater is left in the soft tissue. Every time the student gets anxious again, or stresses himself, or smokes too much, eats poorly, and generally lowers his resistance, another attack can occur. In dentistry, the condition is called A.N.U.G., which stands for acute necrotizing ulcerative gingivitis. It means rapid, frequently painful destruction during the acute phase and a chronic condition thereafter. If you even suspect that you have this, or have had it, see a periodontist for diagnosis and treatment to prevent recurrence.

Even if you're fortunate to not get trench mouth, what else happens in your twenties? If you're not eating well, you may have lowered resistance and lowered repair ability. We said earlier that gingivitis starts progressing when one is thirteen years old. So by twenty, you've had it for a while. Failure to reverse gum inflammation leads to tissue destruction, ultimately reaching the bone. Up until now, while the disease was in the gum, it was still reversible. But now, in your twenties, it may have reached more deeply and begun to dissolve the mineral structure of the bone.

If, in addition, you're not eating well, then you repair more slowly from the bacterial plaque attack. Periodontal disease is treatable, but not reversible. Just because you eat a lot doesn't mean you're well nourished. If your diet isn't balanced, and you're not getting portions of food from each of the four basic food groups, you may be overfed, but undernourished.

To reverse the progress of periodontal disease as much as you can, get into plaque control fast. Start staining, flossing and brushing. Start eating properly. After three weeks, go to your dentist and ask for a complete periodontal examination, including thorough probing, checking for cavities, and taking the necessary X rays to help see the teeth, the bone, and the root areas. The criteria for a good thorough examination will be presented in the next chapter. Naturally, if the dentist recommends treatment, then get it unless you have doubts. If you do have doubts, get a second opinion. But do make a decision after listening to the information, to get as much of your mouth fixed up as you can reasonably afford. If you can't afford much care, go to a hospital clinic or the nearest dental school. Treatment time is slower, but it is done under supervision and the cost is usually low.

If you don't stay with it in your twenties, because nothing bothers you, then by the time you're in your thirties, a small cavity might become such a big one that it actually reaches the nerve. You'll know when this happens because it hurts. Occasionally, a tooth dies without pain, and the nerve degenerates. The breakdown products reach the root tip, and the pressure and infection cause bone around the root tip to dissolve. The infection tries to expand and get out, and when it finishes burrowing through the bone and reaches the soft gum tissue, it causes the gum to expand. This is called an *abscess*.

You may have heard an abscess described as a gum boil or gum pimple. You could have had severe pain during the time it was swelling, or it might not bother you if the abscess breaks open immediately. Usually, there is pain and soreness. The abscess could be a result of infection, in either the gum and bone, or in the nerve and the root of the tooth. Thus it can start from within the tooth, or from the gum space adjacent to the tooth. Go to your dentist as soon as you feel symptoms, let him relieve you, and treat the tooth. *Do not let him extract the tooth.* If he wants to, tell him to just open it up and drain it. After you've had relief, get a second opinion. Most teeth can be saved, if treated properly, as long as there is enough bone remaining around the root of the tooth to give it good support.

So far, things have been going pretty easily. Each dental problem I've proposed has had a clinical symptom. But what about the much more common situation: periodontal disease slowly destroying bone, with no symptoms? With decay, you ultimately feel the problem. Unfortunately, with periodontal disease, you don't until it's frequently too late to treat. That's why it is so important to go to your dentist at least twice a year for examinations and comparisons with your previous visit.

From the twenties on, periodontal examinations should be part of every dental examination. We want to stop periodontal disease as early as possible, because bone can't be replaced easily. It's much better to treat a patient in his twenties for early gum problems than have to do extensive reconstructive periodontal surgery on a patient in his forties. The reason for this is that as more bone is lost, the surgical treatment gets increasingly complicated, and sometimes one has to remove roots, or teeth, or graft bone to rebuild the mouth.

THE THIRTIES—DISEASE IS NOW TAKING ITS TOLL

The Missing Tooth.

By the time a person is in his thirties, several things may have happened. Some of you may have lost a tooth here or there in younger years. Or, if misadvised, you could have lost one recently, because you were told a tooth was beyond repair and you didn't get a second opinion. Lastly, you could have lost a tooth because during treatment, such as a root canal, something happened technically, making it impossible for the dentist to complete the root canal. You might have lost a tooth in an accident, or perhaps even missed one from birth. In any case, you have had a space or spaces in your mouth, and never bothered replacing the missing tooth or teeth because their absence never bothered you. Your appearance was O.K., and you seemed to chew adequately.

What you did not know was that there were shifts and changes occurring in the root and supporting bone of the teeth adjacent to the space.

Shifting and Tilting

Basically, what happens when you lose a tooth, particularly a rear tooth, is that the opposing tooth moves toward the space. This is particularly true of the miss-

SEVEN TEETH ARE AFFECTED BY THE LOSS OR REMOVAL OF ONE TOOTH

ing lower first molar. The upper tooth drops into the space. Teeth next to the space lean in to try to fill it. There are actually seven teeth affected by the loss of the lower first molar.

Periodontal Destruction

As these teeth shift and tilt, they no longer meet correctly while chewing. This puts extra pressure on the bone and periodontal ligament, causing a weakening in these supporting structures. If you have had your periodontal disease developing all along, when the disease reaches the areas of weakened bone and ligament, it progresses very rapidly and the periodontal pocket, with all its bacteria, gets much deeper. Ultimately, as the process accelerates, the deeper the pocket, the more pressure on the tooth from the unbalanced bite. This pressure can actually rock the tooth looser and looser. Finally, when the process has destroyed lots of bone, the tooth is so loose, or abscessing so frequently, that it has to be removed.

Losing the lower first molar thus has a domino effect. If progressive disease continues, when another tooth is lost from decay, or from an accident or periodontal disease, and not replaced, it too affects the remaining teeth. As periodontal disease continues

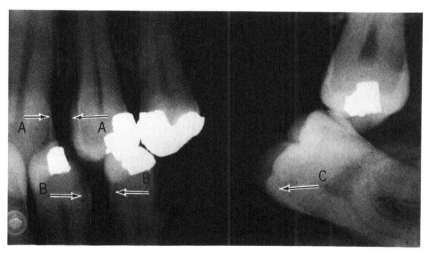

X RAY REVEALING SHIFT AND TILT OF REMAINING TEETH
AFTER THE LOSS OF A TOOTH

and more and more bone is lost, teeth shift, are traumatized during chewing, become loose, and are eventually lost.

If your dentist does not examine you for periodontal problems, and merely suggests replacing the missing tooth with a removable or fixed appliance (like a fixed bridge or partial denture), be concerned. You can't build a mansion on a swamp; you can't build a good bridge on a weak periodontal support.

IMPORTANCE OF THE PERIODONTAL EXAMINATION

The worst mistake you can make is not to have a thorough periodontal examination before undergoing restorative dental treatment as an adult. Restorative treatment may range from anything as simple as fillings, to more complex work such as inlays, onlays, or crowns (described in Chapter 9).

Correct Sequence of Dental Treatment

If you do need periodontal treatment, it should always be done **before** the restorative dentistry, because your gum line may be at a slightly different level after your periodontal treatment. The new dental work must relate to the new gum line. The margin, or edge, of the new dental work should be gently placed just into the new, healthy gum space, or a good bit away from it. It is impossible for a periodontist to treat the gums surgically after restorative dentistry without opening spaces between teeth. If periodontal treatment does create spaces between teeth and restorative dentistry follows, then there is an opportunity to close some of those spaces. That is not possible when treatment is backwards, i.e., doing permanent dental work first and then, within a few years, following with periodontal treatment because of gum problems.

Advantages of Early Periodontal Treatment

Remember this: Although periodontal treatment can stop bone loss, and help save many teeth, it still cannot easily replace structure already lost. Today we graft bone to rebuild some of the lost bone, and transplant gum to restructure tissues in ways we couldn't have clearly envisioned ten years ago. And I expect the next ten years will introduce even more exciting and hopeful ways to rebuild lost structure. But, and it's a big but, these procedures may be costly, possibly painful, and take time. Frequently more extensive dental rebuilding is necessary in a mouth that has undergone periodontal destruction. We have no magic wand to wave to reverse things. And there is no magic mouthwash to use (yet) to eliminate plaque. So please be aware: The earlier you have your mouth probed and the earlier you are treated, the less extensive will be your ultimate therapy, and the less expensive will be your costs. In either case, to maintain your results after periodontal therapy, you still will have to plaque-control. It's the only known way to control the disease, *once the periodontal pockets have been eliminated.*

Why Have Periodontal Surgery?

There has been a great deal of discussion among periodontists, and even in the public media, as to whether periodontal surgery is necessary, when it is, and why. I will expand on the reasons for Periodontal Surgery later in Chapter 10: The Dental Specialties, under "The Periodontist." For the moment, just remember a few facts:

> 1. The two causes of inflammatory periodontal disease are bacterial plaque and your body's hypersensitive reaction to material in the mouth.
> 2. Since the toothbrush bristle and dental floss can get down into the gum space only about 3 mm (a little more than one eighth of an inch), once the gum space is too deep, the disease keeps going on unchecked! This deep gum space is called a pocket and it frequently harbors gum-detaching, bone-destroying bacteria, which brush and floss can't reach, nor can irrigating solutions.
> 3. There have been recent suggestions in the popular press that using an antibiotic, brushing with baking soda and peroxide and irritating with concentrated salt solutions using a Water-Pik can stop periodontal disease, even in the ad-

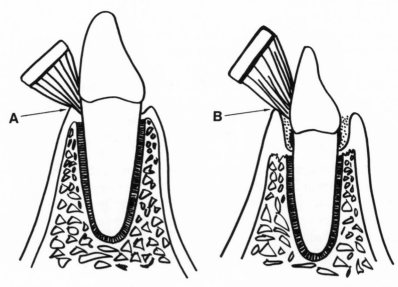

BRISTLES ARE THOROUGHLY
CLEANSING BACTERIAL POCKET

THESE BRISTLES ARE NOT FULLY
ABLE TO CLEANSE THE BACTERIA

vanced stage. There is no definitive proof of this. There have
been no long term follow-ups of patients treated with this
method, and no scientific articles based on carefully designed studies (of large numbers of patients) in the dental literature. As a matter of fact, the deeper the pocket, the less
likely that this method would be effective. For shallow
pockets, it might be of benefit, but so will flossing, brushing,
curetting and root planing. Moreover, when this method is
used in conjunction with antibiotics on a long term basis,
there is a danger of the antibiotic producing resistant bacterial strains in the body, not just the mouth. In addition, over
a long period of time, when the antibiotic is used, there may
be disruption of the bacteria in the small and large intestines. Antibiotics should only be used on a short term basis.
4. Therefore, if your pockets measure deeper than 3 mm
after the shrinkage from plaque controlling for three weeks,
your periodontist must decide whether you can be con-

trolled with further root planing and curettage. If your periodontist feels that the tissue doesn't look as if it will shrink any more with dental treatments (such as curettage or root planing), then at that point, get those gum pockets reduced via a surgical trimming of the excess, unattached, diseased gum wall. Our purpose is for you to have a shallow gum space that you can *easily keep clean!* If at this point your periodontist or dentist suggests you use baking soda, peroxide, and salt water irrigation, at least we're sure it will reach the full depth of the shallow gum space. Pocket elimination is still the tried and true best method for control of the disease, when followed by daily plaque control, according to most dental and periodontal authorities.

5. Finally, follow-up care should include continued monitoring with the phase microscope and video screen to make sure the bacterial infection is not returning. I have been using the microscope now for three years, and it is the most important new tool I have in helping patients control their periodontal disease.

Therefore, if your pockets measure deeper than 3 mm after the shrinkage from plaque controlling for three weeks, and your periodontist feels that the tissue doesn't look as if it will shrink any more with dental treatments (such as curettage or root planing), then at that point, get those gum pockets reduced via a surgical trimming of the excess, unattached, diseased gum wall.

Periodontal Prosthesis

So far, we've discussed periodontal treatment for those of you who have lost bone but still have teeth left saving. There is one more aspect to discuss in terms of dental breakdown and dental repair. That is the area called "periodontal prosthesis" or "periodontal reconstruction." These phrases refer to the joint efforts of a periodontist and a dentist trained in rebuilding broken-down mouths. Sometimes even an orthodontist must be brought in to help reposition teeth before they can be capped and splinted (joined) by the well-trained dentist or prosthodontist. These disciplines, working together in specific sequences of appointments, can help functionally restore some of the most diseased mouths one might imagine. You could lose as much as 75 percent of the bone supporting your teeth, but if you still have a few teeth left, and they are positioned correctly in the mouth, it is still possible for you to avoid dentures. That's the good news.

The bad news is that it costs plenty. In New York City and the surrounding suburbs, it's not uncommon for periodontal treatment on advanced cases to cost in the area of $1,500 to $2,500. The mouth reconstruction, if it's the entire mouth, may range from $9,-000 to $15,000. That's a lot of money for not brushing and flossing early, and not getting examinations and treatment all along. Again, I must stress that it is not good to enter mouth reconstruction—even if you need it and can afford it—without a thorough periodontal examination first. Remember, you could be building a house on quicksand if the gum and bone need treatment and don't get it.

I know of no angrier patients than those referred to me after their dentists have retired, or moved away, or who by accident have gone for an opinion about the state of their gums, *after expensive dental capping was done,* and who are now told, for the first time, that they have lost 50 to 60 percent of their bone, require periodontal surgery, and may have to have some of that beautiful, costly dental work redone! They are furious. They have a right to be. Since dentistry is a blind alley, and the patient has no way of checking one man's opinion except by getting several, it's always a good idea, before making a major investment in your mouth, to double-check.

Just remember, if you're over thirty and faced with such a situation, get that perio-exam before major dental repair. And if you don't need anything major in your thirties, keep getting checked twice a year, and always get probed. That way you are least likely to be one of the growing number of angry people who were fussed with dentally while their bone quietly dissolved away. They got fillings, inlays, caps, or bridges, without ever being made aware of bone destruction.

In conclusion, if you're advised by your dentist or even a periodontist that you just don't have enough bone left around the remaining teeth to save them, again get one or two more opinions before going the denture or implant route. We'll discuss implants at a later time, but one point that I will make now is that your own roots in your own bone are the best implants around. So follow the information you have been given so far, and save your teeth!

SIX
Finding a Good Dentist

THE MOST COMMON method of locating a new dentist is through simple word-of-mouth recommendation. Maybe you've lost a filling, have a toothache, or just don't want to push your luck any further since it's been three years since your last dental visit. So, you ask your best friend: "Who's your dentist? Is he good? Does he hurt?" And your friend replies: "He's great! A very competent dentist and a real nice guy. And he doesn't hurt a bit; he's a doll!" And so you decide to go to your friend's dentist.

Is this the best way to select your new dentist? While a reliable friend's experiences certainly carry weight, it's important to remember that the dentist you choose will be caring for you for many years. The same caution you exercise in choosing a physician, lawyer, psychiatrist or any other trained professional should be used when deciding whose hands you should allow in your mouth.

Ask your friend a few more questions about her dentist: How experienced is he? Does he keep up with the latest advances in dental science? Does he take postgraduate courses yearly to keep up to date? Is he a teacher or lecturer? Is he now, or has he ever been, on a hospital staff or dental school faculty? Teaching is not a guarantee that a dentist will necessarily be skillful or dexterous in the mouth, but it is probable that he will be more careful and current in his approach. The same is true of a dentist who frequently takes postgraduate courses.

If you move to a new city, you may not even know where to begin looking for a good dentist. There are several ways to locate a new dentist without a personal recommendation, and ways to check further on a nonreferred dentist before making the initial appointment.

One very sensible way would be for you to ask your own dentist, before you move, to help you locate a good dentist in the city that will be your new home town. Ask him to look in his A.D.A. directory or call a colleague in that city to try to find someone for you. Very frequently, specialists, particularly periodontists, are in a good position to refer you to a very fine restorative dentist. Endodontists can also be very helpful, since they see the work of many dentists and can usually recognize who is doing superior work and recommend them.

The Yellow Pages will probably be the first place you'll look for a dentist when you're new in town. Not a bad idea, but there are usually a great many doctors listed. Fortunately, there is today a growing subdivision in the listings for general practictioners, specialists, or emergency services. You might also look for the listing of the local dental society. Call the society and express your needs. Every state has an official dental society, and that society has branches or chapters. Tell them your problem and what you want to know: the dentist's office hours, whether foreign languages are spoken, what type of practice he has, if he participates in dental insurance programs, his age range, and so on. It might be helpful to get a list of several names and then call their offices for any further information.

Other helpful sources of information when you are new in town are the teaching universities that have dental schools. Call the administrative offices and ask for information. Of course, you run the risk of getting the answering secretary's favorite dentist, but if you ask for several names, you'll be less likely to have that problem. Again, be sure to specify whether you're looking for a general practitioner or a specialist in a particular field like orthodontics or periodontics.

If there are no dental schools in the area, try contacting a large hospital with a dental staff. The procedure would be the same as in contacting a university. Always get several names and then begin the eliminating process.

All this may take you a day or two of phone work and there's always the possibility that you'll run into a little red tape along the way. But be patient and persevere. The extra time you spend finding a good dentist now could very well save your time and teeth later on.

Personal Preferences

Assuming that you have been resourceful and you now have a list of several dentists obtained either from trusted friends, other medical professionals, the dental society, a university, or hospital, how do you begin the elimination process? You might want to start by considering the following questions:

CONVENIENCE   Is the office located close to work or home? Can you coordinate your schedule with the established office hours? How long is the waiting period for a new patient? What is the policy for emergency treatment?

TYPE OF PRACTICE   Is there just one dentist or are there several? Are they all general practitioners or are there both general practitioners and specialists? Do they perform all services under one roof or do they refer out in special situations? Which of those situations do you prefer? Do you feel it's important to have the same dentist work on you on every visit, and are you willing to sacrifice your personal time to have this arrangement? If not, will you feel comfortable with any member of a reputable practice working on your teeth?

FINANCES   Are you easily able to afford a particular dentist's fee scale? You might ask on the telephone how much a crown or an amalgam filling costs to get an idea of the fee structure. If the dentist is very well recommended, but costly for you, will you be able to work out a manageable payment schedule with the office? If money is extremely tight, would you consider being treated at a clinic facility, or by a competent dental student at a teaching university?

PERSONAL CHOICES   Do you want a dentist in your own age range or do you specifically prefer someone older or younger? Some patients are more comfortable with contemporaries; some prefer someone younger who has been trained more recently; others prefer an older person because of his experience. Do you prefer a male or female dentist? Is it important to you to be treated by someone of the same cultural or religious background? If English is your second language, would you prefer a dentist with whom you could converse in your native tongue?

INSURANCE POLICIES   Find out whether your dentist will prefer you to pay him directly, while you in turn are paid by the insurance company; most dentists prefer this method. He may, however, accept payment directly from the insurance company, with you making up the difference. It is important for you to know this. Read your insurance policy carefully, so that you know any deductibles, limitations, and your benefits. (See also Chapter 15.)

Screening the New Dentist

From the moment of initial contact with the dental office, you should observe how you are treated. Is the secretary warm and courteous on the telephone? Does she ask you whether you are in pain, or what the purpose of your visit is? Does she take a brief history of who referred you, and ask how the dental office can help you? These are some indications of a warm, friendly office, and serve as a reflection of the doctor's personality, training, and directions to his staff.

After you have made your appointment, many offices will send you an office-philosophy letter. This explains what you may expect from the dentist, as well as what he expects of you as a cooperative patient. It might discuss disease prevention, insurance, the goals of complete dentistry, how to keep your mouth healthy in the future, and the like. Usually an office that has gone to the trouble to compose and send such a letter will prove to be thoughtful and well organized in many other areas.

Let us assume now that you have arrived in the dental office for your first appointment. How are you greeted? Do you feel welcomed or are there so many people there that you feel like just another mouth in the crowd?

Are you asked to fill out a medical and dental history form? This is an important prelude to effective dental care, and will let your doctor know whether any special precautions are needed. The dental assistant or doctor should ask whether you have had any history of high or low blood pressure, rheumatic heart disease, diabetes, ulcers, glaucoma, hepatitis, liver or kidney disease, venereal disease,

T.B., alcoholism, drug problems, allergies (especially to medications) cardiovascular disease (including strokes and heart attacks), and any other pertinent information. Some practitioners prefer to take the history in person and some combine the information you filled out with a personal interview. In either case, you definitely should be asked these questions in a thorough interview. Your past history is important for your own protection and optimum treatment, so don't feel that this new dentist is invading your privacy. You should only be offended if he *doesn't* ask for this information from a new patient.

Among the areas you may now want to explore with your new doctor are his philosophies and attitudes toward you and your mouth. If you followed the discussion in Chapter 7, you'll know whether you received a thorough examination. You can also judge whether your problems have been explained well and what the dentist proposes to do to correct them. Interview him carefully regarding whether he tries to save teeth whenever possible. Does he ever refer to specialists for consultation? Does he seem careful, thorough, and concerned?

Next, look around his office. Do you see degrees and certificates indicating activity at professional meetings or courses? Frequently a dentist involved not just with patient care but with active continuing education will receive a certificate for attending a course. He might even be giving a course. This higher level of involvement in dental education doesn't guarantee he'll be a better dentist, but it does show that he's trying to keep current with the latest developments in the field. Finally, find out what his current or past affiliations are, and whether he has any special distinctions in teaching, lecturing or writing.

Notice the kind of patient aids present to help you. Are there pamphlets available that explain various aspects of dental health and disease, or information regarding the periodic need for X rays, or for replacement of missing teeth? Does he have an audio-visual machine so you can watch filmstrips about your mouth, why it breaks down, how to prevent dental disease, and how to repair dental breakdown? Is the staff open to questions you may have about your particular problem, and are they willing to make the office resources available to you?

Is there a phase microscope in the office, to show you your own bacteria under high magnification? If so, not only can you see and directly relate your dental disease to the causative agents, but together you and your dentist can see whether the bacterial types indicate active periodontal disease or a more controlled state of affairs.

Is a hygienist or plaque therapist employed to teach you how to control your own dental disease? To what extent is this new dentist committed not only to repairing your breakdown but making sure it doesn't happen again? Are you going to be repeatedly exposed to the new plaque-control techniques over a few weeks' time so that you can really get into a new skill and modify your former behavior? If you're only going to get a review of brushing and flossing—every three to six months when you come in for a cleaning—then you won't be able to learn the necessary skills well enough, nor are you likely to change your prior dental behavior significantly.

There is another aspect of importance to be considered—the physical environment of the dental office. Do you have the feeling that much thought has been given to creating an environment that is reassuring and comfortable? What do you notice about the dental equipment in the room? Does it seem modern? Are most of the instruments and drills hidden from view or easily seen? Is the room where you will receive your dental treatment cheery, or is it depressing and somber? Is it very clean, or is it dirty or disarrayed? Is there background music to help you relax? Zero in on how you feel about this room in which you will receive treatment. Do you feel comfortable and at ease here, or does it make you nervous and upset?

How many treatment rooms are there? It is very hard to render a preventive service, in addition to a reparative service, unless there are at least two rooms. The second room is needed for a hygienist or plaque-control therapist, to train you and work with you as you acquire the skills to remove bacteria in your mouth.

Now for the most important issue of all. Assuming that the dentist has satisfied you on most of these issues, how do you like him? Is he warm, empathetic, patient? Does he give you the feeling of being knowledgeable as he explains the various findings of the dental examination to you? Do you feel reassured and, finally, do you trust him?

Is he reasonably good at listening? Remember, he's a dentist, not a psychiatrist, so don't ask him everything under the sun. Try to restrict your questions to honest, sincere ones about your mouth. Find out if he thinks any breakdown has occurred and what he proposes to do about it.

If you're afraid to ask him these or any other questions, there's a problem in the relationship. It's most important that you feel free to ask him anything about your care and treatment. Get everything explained clearly, and in language you can understand.

Take notes. Make sure he presents a coherent treatment plan, and that you understand all aspects of it. Find out approximately how long it will take to correct your problems. *If, at the time of consultation, you think substantial cost may be involved, have your spouse present if such financial issues are usually jointly discussed.* It is almost impossible for one mate to be given a dental diagnosis and accurately relate the findings and fees to the other mate. Too many important details or nuances may be left out, which may make a big difference in how each person feels about the money to be spent for treatment.

If there are any residual questions, always feel free to request a second, short consultation to discuss problem areas or lingering doubts. You should feel perfectly comfortable about who is going to treat you and what you will pay for those services.

If the dentist is preventively oriented, you may actually feel his enthusiasm and so become enthusiastic yourself. And you *should* feel excited about getting control of your dental health, perhaps for the first time, by controlling the cause of disease ... bacterial plaque. You are now a partner and co-therapist in the dental health arena. Remember—prevention saves money, saves time, and saves teeth!

SEVEN

Dental Costs and Why They Vary

THROUGHOUT THE U.S., there are major differences in fees for the same service. By major, I mean a variation of 50 to 100 percent. Are these differences justified by higher levels of education on the part of the dentists rendering care, or are they a result of charging what the traffic will bear? To what degree does a fee reflect a man's ego, his fear of rejection, his conscience, his community price level? To what degree does it involve his patient's ability to pay, and his patient's dental needs? As you see, there are many considerations that go into the establishment of a fee.

Let's analyze the situation from several viewpoints to create a total picture. To start with, the dentist is in business. He is in a service business taking care of people's teeth, and being paid for his time, judgment, and skill. He is also paid for the materials and appliances he makes or inserts, and the services other members of his staff may render in supporting the dental care he offers.

Overhead

The dentist has certain overhead costs which go into his final fee to you. These costs include staff salaries, rent, supplies, utilities, telephone, accounting, legal, laundry, equipment maintenance, replacement, stationery, bookkeeping and billing, conventions and continuing education courses, dues and subscriptions, laboratory bills, and so on.

When all these are taken together, they represent the cost to the dentist of being in business of caring for people's teeth and oral structures. The costs may be figured annually, and then broken down into monthly or weekly figures. A dentist may find that it costs him $50,000 or $100,000 a year to run his practice. It is the amount that he earns above that figure that will represent his profit, which is usually his salary.

For these reasons of overhead, it should be obvious that if you pay $1,000 for dental work, he may retain only $450 of that before taxes. After city, state, and federal taxes, he may retain only 20 to 25 percent of the fee you paid him. So when thinking about his fee, please remember he only gets to keep a fraction of it.

Educational Differences

As a general rule, specialists will charge somewhat more (perhaps 20 percent) than a general dentist will for a comparable procedure. For that difference in fee, you are paying for the extra years of training and education that the specialist acquired to become an expert in a certain dental discipline. Today, most specialty programs for periodontics, orthodontics, endontics, prosthodontics, etc. are for two years beyond dental school. In addition, there may be an internship involved. During those years the dental specialist-to-be is earning poorly. He may be twenty-eight to thirty years old before he finally gets into private practice and starts to earn a living for himself and his family. These lost years of income are somewhat compensated for by his broader and deeper knowledge of his dental specialty. His experience with the nuances of diagnosis and treatment usually result in a more complete, and superior, treatment. Many problems do not require his services. There are many problems that should be treated by the general dentist. Usually the general dentist will make the decision regarding the need for a specialist. Conversely, you may realize you would rather be diagnosed and treated by a specialist for a certain condition or situation. If so, be prepared for a fee differential for the specialist's additional education and training to provide the best one can receive.

What about the differences between general practitioners? They do exist. Does education bear on these differences? Possibly so. If the dentist takes quite a few postgraduate courses for which he pays, and which also require that he give up productive office time and perhaps private time, somehow he has to be compensated for the additional training he is acquiring to service you more completely. He is entitled to pass on that cost to his patients in his fee for those services.

It may be possible that his talent and skill allow him to perform a service better. Here too, final results count. If the general practitioner consistently performs a better service than his peers for certain procedures, he may correctly feel that he should be paid for his expertise, just as he would be as a specialist.

The Community in Which the Dentist Practices

Here we have a very significant factor in fee differential. There are traditions in a community. Suburban communities tend to be more homogenous than metropolitan centers. Peer pressure and fear of losing patients frequently keep fees within a community fairly close to one another.

One new element that is changing the fee differential is the advertising dentist. Usually, dentists who advertise have larger facilities, which are geared to servicing many people. They employ many types of dentists, but in my own checking of these facilities, I found that most dentist-employees are either just out of school, or trying to start their practice and working for the advertising facility part time to earn extra income. Another frequent type of employee is an older dentist who has decided that he would rather have a definite patient flow, and a guaranteed salary, than worry about how nice a guy he is, or how he can keep building his practice.

These advertising centers usually offer dental care at fees below the private dental community levels. Generally, one gets what one pays for. If crowning (capping) is being offered at 40 percent less than the usual community fee, that difference has to be paid for by less attention to detail in preparing the tooth for the crown (cap), and in the laboratory work that goes into the fabrication of the crown.

Standards may have to be lower, because dentistry is an art as well as a science. Art requires tremendous attention to detail. One cannot mass-produce art. Similarly, one cannot mass-produce excellent crown and bridge work (capping) or mass-produce surgical work.

One can produce less complicated service, use less expensive materials, and employ cheaper labor. Prices will then be lower, but so will quality. You get what you pay for. Needless to say, each advertising dental center must be evaluated on its own merits, including satisfied patients.

There are several dental centers, as well as union facilities, that offer "gum treatment." As should now be evident by our earlier discussion of periodontal treatment, there is no such thing as true "gum treatment" in the manner in which it is being promoted. Either you have periodontal pockets or you don't. If you do, you'll need either definitive root planing and curettage to shrink the pockets, or surgical elimination of the pockets. If they are shallow, root planing followed by curettage may be sufficient. For many adults, surgical pocket elimination will be necessary. But these treatment approaches require great skill, care, and time. The "gum treatments" offered in the advertising facilities are frequently just "cleanings"—in which the teeth are cleaned, usually just slightly into the gum space, and the gum poked a little. One must raise serious questions as to whether any real, lasting improvement can occur from such an approach. Studies by the Norwegian investigator Waerhaug very clearly showed that superficial cleaning would still leave plaque, calculus, and disease, and that pockets deeper than 3 mm become very difficult to keep thoroughly bacteria-free. As the pockets get deeper, periodontal destruction increases. Therefore, one must be probed, and a decision must be made as to what course of treatment would get the gum spaces back to a shallow depth that you could control yourself with flossing and brushing. It is you who should be giving yourself daily gum treatment on a mouth that is periodontally healthy with no pockets.

Your Ability to Pay As It Relates to Your Dental Needs

The majority of adults may need greater or lesser amounts of dentistry, depending on the eyes of the beholder, namely, the particular dentist examining and diagnosing. In turn, his ability to diagnose will depend on his level of training, the courses he has taken, whether other dentists see his work (as happens in a group practice or where he works with a periodontist), or whether he is a law unto himself in his own office with no other professional ever seeing the quality of his work.

Sometimes older practitioners like to fall back on their years of experience in trying to advise a patient. In many situations, their experience, coupled with continuing education, gives them a seasoned approach. However, one can also repeat the same errors for thirty years, and indeed have thirty years of experience! So mere experience, or age, is not the only criterion in evaluating a mouth. Experience plus continuing education is crucial!

A patient should be able to judge, by the care, detail of the examination, and thorough explanation of the treatment plan, why a particular approach is being recommended. A fee should be given that seems fair to the dentist for the time, energy, and effort to be expended in obtaining the desired result. In the event that the best treatment plan appears too costly, a modified treatment plan should be given, and also discussed and compared with the first plan.

Second Opinion

I think that given the variation in fees within a community, your own intuition and intelligence should allow you to determine, should you go for a second opinion, which dentist and which plan make more sense to you. The follow-up care, and the continued training in disease prevention and checking for any new breakdown, all form part of the type of care you would find most beneficial. Since this is a long-term investment and a long-term relationship, a higher fee for the right service should not be a deterrent. The extra difference, in fact, may be compared to insurance, which saves you future repair bills.

Special Items Entering Into the Fee Involving Overhead

QUALITY OF THE DENTAL SUPPORT TEAM   People don't usually work for nothing, and for the dentist to have a pleasant, hard-working, loyal, efficient staff requires a great deal of energy, time, and skill on everyone's part. The time spent in building a dental team is above and beyond regular work hours. It costs money to produce a well-coordinated team. It has been estimated that training a new person may cost $5,000 the first year in doctor's time and staff time, beyond that person's salary. Yet a friendly, efficient staff is very important in your feeling comfortable and welcome in the dentist's office. The smooth functioning of a well-run office is for your benefit. It's not an accident, but a result of careful hiring, good training, good salaries, and good benefits. If not well compensated, a well-trained staff member won't stay. Therefore, entering into the cost of your work is the dentist's cost in building a well-trained staff, even if it's a small staff.

COST OF LABORATORY WORK   One major area for the general dentist or prosthodontist that is not usually present for the other specialists is the extensive cost of the dental laboratory work. This includes the bill to the dentist for crowns, onlays, inlays, bridges, partial dentures, complete dentures, and so on. These costs can be a very substantial part of the dentist's overhead, and the better the quality of the laboratory's work, the more they will charge for it. Laboratory work, like dental work, is an art. As laboratories are forced to turn out more and more work, they must have a fall-off in quality. As they attempt to mass-produce, the product suffers. Your dentist may have higher fees for his work, but he may be using one of the better laboratories in your area, in order to get a superior product for you. Ask him about this, and find out how he feels about different dental laboratories. If he says they're all the same, be suspicious. If he takes great pride in the one he works with, he's probably using a higher standard for the work he's placing in your mouth, and so is his laboratory. Be thankful you have chosen wisely.

EFFICIENCY   Another very important area for consideration is the efficiency of the dentist and his team. Certain dentists have studied how they themselves work, and how others work. They have found out where they duplicated procedures or wasted time, and have tried to eliminate these nonproductive areas. This is called "time-and-motion study," and is used in many fields. By eliminating waste time, dentists have increased their productivity with no sacrifice of quality. In turn, they may be able to offer you a lesser fee for the identical service someone else may offer you. So you gain because of their efficiency, and they do too.

COLLECTIONS   You directly influence your dentist's fees by how you pay your bills. If your dentist has a definite arrangement with you, and you do not bring or send your monthly payment to him on time, it becomes necessary for his secretary either to contact you by phone or send you another bill. All of this costs money—for the labor, materials, and postage. Adding all of this together for all patients in a practice easily costs several thousand dollars a year. Since this is part of the office overhead, the dentist must pass this cost on to you. Therefore, you can do your part to reduce these unnecessary costs by paying promptly, or by letting the secretary know if your financial situation has changed. New arrangements can then be made without unnecessary embarrassment or avoidance.

Similarly, if you have insurance, you can save the secretary time by filling in as much as you can on the insurance forms. Not only will this reduce overhead, which will come back to you in lower fees, but the secretary will appreciate your consideration, and when you need special courtesy, will be much more likely to give attention to your area of need. Just remember, as in any area of human affairs, it's a two way street: to the extent that you help, you will be helped.

To summarize our discussion, let's remember the following:

1. Make sure that you know, in writing, what dental services you have contracted for, how much their cost will be, and what your financial payments will be.

2. If you have insurance, you should know whether your obligation is to pay the dentist, while the insurer is to pay you, or whether the dentist will directly accept the insurance payment, with you making up the difference.

3. Try to strive for quality care.

4. Fees can differ by 20 percent and still be fair, and that a specialist will charge somewhat more than a general dentist.

5. The dentist is also in business as he provides health care. If he is a poor businessman, he will go bankrupt and be forced to stop practice. He is entitled to a fair return for his years of education, skill, patience, and judgment.

6. If you treat your dentist with respect, you will most likely be treated similarly.

7. If you have a comprehensive treatment plan, ask questions

to understand why certain types of treatment are being recommended.

8. Make sure you have good rapport, as this type of relationship could be a long one.

9. In the final analysis, it is not the fee, but the quality and excellence of care, that is most important.

EIGHT

What You Should Know About a Good Dental Examination

NOW WE ARE GETTING into some nitty-gritty, the real essentials of how to know what you're getting. Now you know how you got into trouble, where it leads, and how to get your children correctly launched on their good dental-health trip. But, since you don't live in a dental vacuum, you have to relate somehow, somewhere, to a careful, progressive, well-educated and well-informed guardian of your teeth and periodontium. Where do we find such a dentist? (Or, perhaps you are already under the care of one.)

I will list for you what I consider to be a thorough dental examination. I will also tell you what you should look for, and why. When we finish, you should understand the basic areas, and be able to decide whether you have been getting a thorough examination, as well as how to evaluate a new dentist.

THE VISUAL EXAMINATION

Soft-Tissue Exam

THE CANCER EXAM   Ten percent of the cancers of the body occur in the mouth. Therefore, it is important to be examined in the following areas: lips, cheeks, mucous membranes, palate, throat, oropharynx, undersurface of the tongue, and the floor of the mouth. Lymph nodes under the lower jaw and alongside the neck should be felt to see if they are enlarged. If so, it may be a result of present or past upper-respiratory infections, or current infections of another nature. It may also indicate something more serious. Your dentist should check these areas and advise you of his findings.

GINGIVA AND MUCOUS MEMBRANE   These tissues should be checked for inflammation, abscesses, abrasions, growths, swelling, bleeding sores, or ulcers. All findings should be recorded, and you should be asked how long you have had the problem and whether it recurs.

Facial-Structure Exam

The outside of the face should be examined from a direct frontal view for lack of symmetry, such as an overdeveloped jaw or underdeveloped group of muscles, which might indicate potential or actual problems in speech or chewing, or perhaps a benign or malignant tumor.

Palpation for Sore Chewing Muscles

When this visual inspection is complete, your dentist should feel the area inside the mouth on each side of the lower jaw behind the last molar teeth. He is checking where a band of tissue called a *raphe* inserts and runs from the upper to the lower jaw. Several of the chewing muscles insert here, and tenderness to finger pressure may reveal muscle spasm due to disturbances in your bite.

If the dentist does notice something in any of the above areas of inspection, he should make a written notation. Then he can decide on a course of action, if needed, or have a guideline with which to compare on a future examination.

Gingival Examination

Next, he should look at the gum (gingiva) and see whether it is pink or red, inflamed, puffy, or normal and flat; whether any recession has occurred, and whether the gum band is wide enough to prevent recession. The dentist looks to see if any muscle-pull from the mucous membrane is causing recession. He marks all this information down.

Mouth Cleanliness

Next he observes your mouth cleanliness or lack of it. Is there a heavy coating of plaque, a moderate amount, or none? Is there heavy tartar formation, particularly on the lower anterior teeth, or on the cheek side of the upper posterior teeth? How about stain? Is it from smoking?

Saliva

How about the saliva? Is it watery, or thick and slimy? More bacteria generally grow in thick, ropy saliva.

Decay, Broken Fillings, Removable Appliances

Is there a generalized condition of decay, or chipping, or erosion near the neck of the teeth? Are there removable dental appliances? How well do they fit? Do the dental restorations look new or old? Are they carefully done, or was the work sloppy? All this is written down.

The Bite

Next, the dentist examines the bite itself. He checks to see whether the teeth hit evenly when you close your jaws. He does this with ribbons or very fine strips of paper, or film coated with special marking materials. Then he lets you slide out your lower jaw in several directions, with the marking material placed in the upper and lower teeth. He sees if you have high spots occurring on the surface of one or a few teeth when the teeth come into contact. He records the information. He checks the lateral movements of the jaw and the straight slide forward of the lower front teeth against the upper front teeth, and finally he checks to see if any rear teeth touch on the opposite side from the side to which he directs your jaw to move. From all this information, he knows how your bite works and whether it needs any bite correction, or perhaps any building up of certain teeth that don't meet opposing teeth. He can also take study models, so that he has a permanent hard-plaster model of your teeth. He can even take a spatial relationship of your upper jaw to your head, and your lower jaw to the upper jaw, so that he can study how your jaw closes. He does this on a special machine, to help analyze the bite. This is not always needed, but is very helpful if much rebuilding of the bite is going to be done.

The Temporomandibular Joint (TMJ)

Next, he examines the joints on each side near the ear. He checks for popping or clicking when you open and close, and tries to correlate that with any history of pain or limited ability in mouth opening. He feels the chewing muscles to see if there is any tenderness, and asks whether you have many headaches, stiff necks, or other problems with the chewing muscles or joints, that you have noticed. This helps him determine whether you have temporomandibular joint dysfunction, and whether it requires treatment. Most cases of TMJ pain are related to disharmonies in the bite (the way the teeth meet and chew). The dentist will have to put all this information together to know how to treat you if it's needed.

THE PERIODONTAL EXAMINATION

Open Contacts

Now we get to the periodontium. The first thing the dentist would want to know is whether there are any loose or sloppy contacts between teeth, where foods wedge.

He can test for this with dental floss. If the floss passes through too easily, with no resistance or snap, or if he doesn't have to slide it back and forth to pass the tooth contact, then the contact is too loose. He writes down all open contacts. These must be corrected later to prevent food wedging between teeth.

Charting Pockets and Mobility

Next he moves to the periodontal examination itself.

The key to this exam is recording all the information so as to have a permanent record. The dentist's assistant should write down all the missing teeth, and the dentist should then examine each side of each tooth, in the gum space, with a periodontal probe. This gum-space reading is most important: It helps determine whether any surgery is needed, and what kind. Numbers higher than 3 indicate the need for some treatment to reduce pocket depth. Depending on the type of tissue, it might be treated with curettage, or it might need some form of gum surgery. Each reading is permanently recorded. As the patient, you might hear a series of numbers, like "six . . . three . . . six, five . . . two . . five." When all pockets (the deepened gum spaces) have been measured, the dentist checks the looseness or tightness of the tooth. He calls this "mobility," and his assistant records this.

DENTAL EXAMINATION

Last, after finishing his periodontal exam, the dentist does a clinical examination of the teeth. He checks for cavities, broken teeth, broken fillings, erosion, and cavities next to old fillings.

The X Ray Examination

This information is correlated with the X rays, which should include films showing all the roots of the teeth, as well as clear views in between teeth where they contact each other. For my complete examinations, I like an X-ray set of twenty films. Probably, one might vary between sixteen and twenty-two films to get totally accurate information, but not less. The reason for this many films is that the dentist needs to see clearly the following areas: all root tips, the sinuses, the bone around the teeth and behind the last teeth, and the contacts between all teeth. A full examination with this number of X rays should be done approximately every thirty-six months. At six-month intervals, for periodic checks, four bitewing X rays will suffice. They will show any new cavities but will not show the root tips or bone well. Shown below are three X rays illustrating mild, moderate, and advanced periodontal disease. Another X ray shows a deep cavity under a crown.

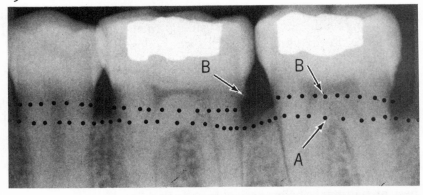

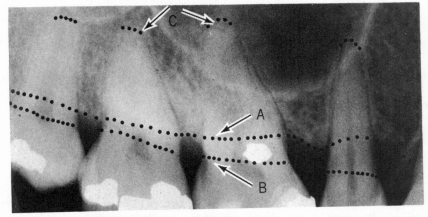

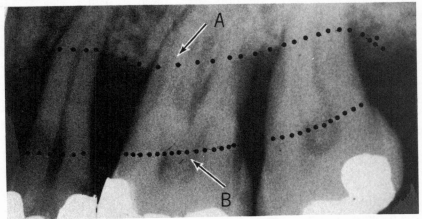

X RAYS OF MILD, MODERATE, AND SEVERE PERIODONTAL DISEASE

DEVELOPING THE TREATMENT PLAN

By correlating the X rays and the number readings of the gum space, the dentist should be able to determine which teeth have lost too much bone to be saved, which teeth can be saved but definitely require treatment, and which teeth have a normal bone and normal gum space.

If the dentist recognizes a periodontal problem, he should decide, in all honesty, whether his training would permit him to completely eliminate the pockets and correct any problems in the bone, either via sculpting or bone-grafting techniques. It is difficult to treat moderate to advanced cases of periodontal disease and get really good results unless one has had thorough training in periodontics. Many dentists have had introductory courses in periodontal therapy, but these courses do not make one a periodontist. There is much more to diagnosing and evaluating a case of periodontal breakdown than just measuring pockets. One has to join together all the available diagnostic information, including diet history, type of bacteria present, occlusion of the teeth, any contributing conditions like diabetes or other medical health problems; evaluate the number of teeth remaining, their root length supported by bone, what type of dental restoration will be needed following periodontal treatment, and so on. Moreover, the dentist must decide whether his surgical training will allow him to get an optimum surgical result, and whether he and his staff can successfully motivate the patient to control his plaque.

I feel that dentists who have recently graduated, and who have had training at their universities with a reasonable number of surgical cases, might undertake simpler periodontal cases with pocket depth no deeper than 5 or 6 mm. and with no involvement between the roots of molar teeth. Similarly, dentists in practice for quite a while who have taken postgraduate courses in periodontal surgery—where they had direct surgical experience under supervision on at least four patients—should be able to undertake the simpler periodontal procedures. But those dentists who have not had a good deal of surgical experience and have simply had lecture courses should not, in my opinion, undertake to operate periodontally on patients, without further study and practice under the supervision of an experienced periodontist. It simply is not fair to you, the patient, because it frequently means failure, and may subject you to surgery a second time or, worse, make you lose the involved tooth or teeth. And this can happen from misdiagnosis as well as from poor surgical technique.

In addition, the more difficult a case gets, the more considerations have to be raised regarding long-term success. Let's say that you are the patient. It's important to know whether you are able and willing to do plaque control daily. Without your daily cooperation, your results after treatment could really slip, and your periodontal condition might begin to come back. I cannot stress this too strongly. If you do have surgery done, make sure the dental office is monitoring you with the phase microscope after completion of active treatment. A patient who has had periodontal disease is still susceptible to it even after treatment. To prevent recurrence, you must stain and remove plaque daily. You must see your dentist or periodontist every few months (this could vary from one month to six months) to allow him to reprobe and make sure there is no return of pocket depth or bleeding points, and to remove any tartar (calculus) that has formed, and to be checked with the microscope.

We'll expand more on how to get healthy and keep healthy periodontally, after treatment, in Chapter 10. For now, let's return to our thorough dental examination. When your dentist has completed his soft tissue examination, joint examination, bite examination, periodontal examination, and X-ray examination, he is able to put together your ideal treatment plan.

TREATMENT PRIORITIES

This treatment plan will probably be very comprehensive, and have your best interests at heart. The dentist will discuss the elimination of any infections, removal of hopeless teeth, whether or not you require periodontal treatment or root-canal treatment, and so on. He will also discuss your bite, and what type of dental restorations or replacements you may need. He may recommend bridgework, or connecting teeth together with a process called splinting, if your teeth are loose. We'll discuss all of these special procedures in Chapter 10 (Dental Specialties).

In summary, he should explain what you need, why you need it, what the cost will be, and what choices you have. If he's good, and if you've never had this type of thorough examination before, you'll learn a great deal. Hopefully, if you've read this book, you should be able to ask some pretty sharp questions, and get satisfactory answers.

You may find that the initial treatment plan is too costly. This frequently happens. Ask the dentist for one or two alternate plans, costing less, that would still attend to the most important needs. Also ask him if he were to proceed more slowly with the ideal treatment plan, how long it would take to complete treating your mouth. Now consider each of the three possibilities, in terms of long-term value and cost:

1. Ideal treatment plan done within one year.
2. Ideal treatment done over two or three years
3. Alternate plan—less costly

List on a piece of paper the advantages or disadvantages of each. Narrow down to your two best choices. If you have more questions at that point, recheck with the dentist. Then go to your best choice and get started.

If for any reason you cannot afford any plan, seek a second opinion. If it confirms the first opinion, then your two financial alternatives would be to go either to a dental university or a hospital clinic near you. If you've listened carefully to the dentist's diagnosis and recommendations, and *have written them down for study,* you should know, when you go to a university or clinic, whether you are getting treated properly. Costs will be less there, but the work may not be as well done by the students or young graduates as they would be by an experienced dentist. Conversely, under proper supervision it might be better! Obviously, you will spend much more time at a clinic or university than at a private office. So you must decide what your time and inconvenience is worth as opposed to the cost saving. Then you do whichever is better for your circumstances.

Two final recommendations. First, if the dentist you are going to, or are thinking of going to, does not stress prevention, including plaque control and diet evaluation, or if you continue to have lots of decay, loosening teeth, or bleeding gums, look elsewhere. He's practicing in the past, not the present.

Second, beware of the dentist who claims he can do everything well. There are a few geniuses around who are brilliant, both diagnostically and technically, but they are very rare.

So, if you have a periodontal condition that is moderate to severe (pockets of 6 to 9 mm), get to a good periodontist. If you need root-canal work, and your dentist has done a lot of root canals, he would be fine for your problems. But if you don't think he's highly experienced, go to a root-canal specialist. If your dentist wildly resists your going for second opinions, gets defensive, or feels threatened, chances are that he's not that confident of his diagnostic or technical abilities. He should respect your feelings and desire to make the right decision. Think carefully about him. Your relationship with your dentist is usually a long-term one. You both want to be comfortable with each other. Talk to him about your feelings, what you hope to get from his office, and his dental care, why you want to prevent disease and be helped in that direction. Give him a chance to cooperate and to grow with you if he has fallen a little behind the times.

But if you find that he's uncooperative, defensive, or says that preventing disease is nonsense (and that tooth loss is inevitable), then cut out fast! Do not walk, but run, to someone more current with today's knowledge, and who is more open minded.

As a final checklist, here's what should have been done during a thorough examination:

1. Soft tissue, face and neck exam—outside the mouth
2. Soft-tissue exam inside the mouth
3. Joint and chewing muscles exam
4. Bite exam
5. Periodontal exam with pocket measuring and recording
6. X-ray examination
7. Cavity check
8. The consultation, summing up all the above information, with treatment and recommendations, including alternative choices

NINE

How Teeth Are Repaired, Including Full Mouth Reconstruction

SEQUENCE OF TREATMENT

In Chapter 7 we discussed what a thorough oral and dental examination included. We said that wherever possible, the ideal treatment plan is the best plan for you. Obviously, since it is the most thorough, and usually recommends dental materials that will last longest without breaking or causing other dental problems, this plan may be the most costly. But before focusing on dental repair, let's go over the sequence of treatment you should expect if you are with a new dentist or have not seen your regular dentist for more than a year.

After he or she completes a very thorough examination as outlined in the preceding chapter, let us imagine the following discussions, with the findings and recommendations you might hear:

1. Your oral tissues do not present any abnormal lesions or growths. You do not indicate any possibility of having oral cancer, and you certainly do not require a biopsy.

2. You have one (or more) teeth so badly decayed, and periodontally weakened, that extraction is recommended for the tooth or teeth. Make sure *you* ask whether they could be saved with root canal, or with periodontal treatment. If you are told the teeth can't be saved, you might consider getting a second opinion, unless it's obvious to you after discussion with the dentist why they can't be saved. If you do have extractions, always discuss how the missing teeth will be replaced, and what the costs will be. Once you have the whole picture, you can make an intelligent decision.

After advising you regarding any extractions, your dentist will consider any infection present. In examining for endodontic or periodontal infection, your dentist is considering two possibilities:

Endodontic Infection

You may have infection at the bottom of a root. This may be seen on the X ray as a darkened, diffuse area. You may have told the dentist you have pain on taking anything hot or cold in your mouth. He may see a cavity in the tooth giving you these symptoms. In studying your X rays, he might see a dark area on the side or on the tip of your root, with a thin white line encircling the dark area. This would be a cyst.

If he finds any of the above, he will recommend root-canal treatment, *assuming there is enough bone around the tooth root to make the tooth worth keeping.* Ask him whether the tooth has enough bone support, because if it has also had periodontal breakdown, and is loose, and has less than 25 percent bone support, it usually should be removed.

Let's assume that the bone-support level is good. The dentist has recommended that you have root-canal treatment. What should you know?

1. Root canals eliminate the infection in most cases. Chances for success are high.

2. You should be told the *cost* of root canal treatment by the one who will do it. Your dentist may do the root-canal work, or he may refer you to a specialist—an endodontist—who only does root-canal work.

3. *You should also be told that treatment does not usually end just with root-canal work itself.* Usually, because the tooth gets brittle after the nerve is removed by the root-canal treatment, a *crown* is recommended to prevent fracture of the tooth. Usually, it is also necessary to have a *post* inserted in the tooth before crowning, to make it strong. All these extra recommendations, and more complete treatment, will also cost extra money. Therefore, you should know the total cost of saving the tooth before receiving the root-canal treatment. *Saving a tooth with good bone support is still preferable to extracting it and replacing the missing tooth with a bridge.*

4. If there is some chance of failure, you should also be advised of the likelihood. Obviously, in many situations the dentist cannot guarantee the success of treatment without actually treating, but if he has his doubts and yet is willing to try, find out his feelings regarding likelihood of a successful result, and what his dental recommendations would be if you preferred to extract the tooth.

Periodontal Infection—Are Your Teeth Losing Their Bone Support?

Peridontal infection is frequently less obvious to the patient and yet, as I have explained, is present in almost all adult mouths. It is diagnosed most accurately by careful *probing* and microscopic bacterial examination, and further clarified by careful interpretation of well-taken X rays, which show the bone surrounding the roots. If the X rays are distorted, overdeveloped, or underdeveloped, or do not include a picture of the complete root with surrounding bone, they should be retaken. *A poor X ray is no X ray at all; X-rays should be of diagnostic quality.*

By using the probe, the X ray, and checking for tooth looseness, the dentist can determine how much periodontal disease exists. He can also tell whether the disease in different areas of the mouth is in an active or more resting stage. You can help him by telling him of any pain, swelling, abscesses, or other problems that you have noticed.

When he has completed your entire periodontal examination, and also examined your *bite,* the number of *missing teeth,* how many remaining *roots* are present and where they are located, the condition of your *present dental work,* whether *decay* is present that will require new dental work or redoing of old work, and correlated this information with your state of *health,* medically and emotionally, he is ready to make his recommendations.

He can now tell you which teeth don't have enough bone present to justify retaining. These teeth may have abscessed in the past, or may be very likely to cause infection in the near future. Usually, teeth with less than 25 percent bone support, or with bone loss in between and around molar roots, don't offer much hope for long-term retention. Upper molars do worse than lower molars.

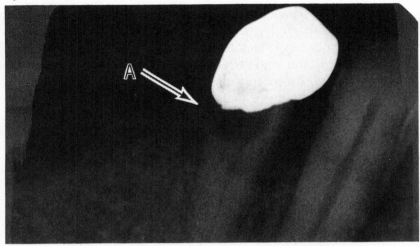

THIS X RAY REVEALS NEW DECAY UNDER AN EXISTING FILLING

Each situation must be related individually, with respect to your age, the number of remaining teeth, any systematic diseases like diabetes, and your own interest in keeping your remaining teeth free of plaque. If saving a tooth or teeth seems extremely questionable, it is usually best to remove them before the infection surrounding them causes destruction of the bone on an adjacent tooth. Over-retention of periodically diseased teeth frequently leads not just to loss of the worst tooth, but of several others. This happens because the periodontal infection can spread to the adjacent tooth. Again, if in doubt about saving or extracting a tooth or teeth, consult another dentist or a periodontist for a second opinion, or two periodontists in case your dentist's opinion differs from that of the first periodontist.

We will discuss how periodontal treatment actually is performed in the chapter on the dental specialties (Chapter 10).

For the moment, let's just say that under the *ideal treatment plan,* you would try to save all teeth that are retainable and would eliminate periodontal infection by:

1. Learning plaque control.
2. Having your teeth and roots cleaned above and below the gum line as thoroughly as possible.

3. Where pocket depth is greater than 3 mm, having periodontal treatment done to reduce or eliminate the pockets, assuming that there is adequate bone support around the tooth. (With adequate bone support, we don't want any pockets. With less than 35 percent remaining bone support, there might be a compromise regarding the final depth of the pocket.) There are several different approaches to pocket elimination, based on recognition of the type of gum tissue being treated, as well as other clinical considerations. This will be completely discussed in Chapter 9.

4. After completing periodontal therapy and any necessary root-canal treatment, you would then follow through on the dental restorative plan. Restorative dentistry is usually designed to stabilize loose teeth, replace missing teeth, even out the bite so that upper and lower teeth can effectively chew against each other, and, last but not least, provide a pleasant, natural-looking smile and normal speech patterns.

THE DENTAL TREATMENT PLAN

Ideal Treatment Plans

The objective of the ideal treatment plan is to try to save all teeth that are worth saving for as long as possible. To do this correctly, you might need root-canal treatment, periodontal treatment, and comprehensive dental treatment.

In dental circles, the phrase "full-mouth reconstruction," or "full-mouth rehabilitation," refers to the ideal dental treatment plan. Technically speaking, even just restoring a few teeth to their ideal form and function is mouth rehabilitation, but the term usually refers to the more comprehensive case. It requires, in most cases, coordination of the endodontic specialist, the periodontist, and sometimes the orthodontist, and then—coordinating the results of all of the above—the dentist or prosthodontist.

One of the differences between a dentist and a prosthodontist is based on training. A prosthodontist today usually has had either two additional years of special training in the area of fixed and removable dental appliances, or, by virtue of his continuing education, has taken and passed certain examinations, which acknowledge him as being duly qualified to present himself to the public as a prosthodontist.

This does not mean that a dentist, if well trained, could not undertake mouth reconstruction. But it does mean that mouth reconstruction is very complicated and requires excellent diagnostic judgment and great technical skill to obtain a result that is not only functional, esthetic, and comfortable, but will preserve the remaining teeth. It does mean that, if in doubt, considering the costs involved (these could range from $8,000 to $15,000 for a complete mouth reconstruction), you should get more than one opinion. Speak to other satisfied patients, and try to determine the qualifications of the dentist you are considering. Discuss his prior training in mouth reconstruction to help you determine whether he is best qualified to undertake the complex task of rebuilding your mouth.

Let's now discuss what is involved in rebuilding a mouth so that you can fully appreciate what modern dentistry can accomplish, and how much thought and planning is involved.

Rebuilding Your Mouth

When the diagnosis is made that you require full mouth reconstruction, you are entering a new experience of high cost and lengthy visits at various dental offices, with the need for patience on your part. That sounds unpleasant, but the results are worth it. It took many years for your mouth to break down to its present sorry state. It's really quite an accomplishment to restore your mouth to a healthful, functioning, and esthetically pleasing state in the twelve to eighteen months usually needed.

How is it done? Usually, the dentist or prosthodontist confers with a periodontist to establish a treatment plan. They then discuss this plan with you to make sure that it meets your approval regarding the cost and length of time it will take to rebuild your mouth. Occasionally, the other specialties, such as orthodontics and endodontics (root-canal work), are needed. Orthodontics is employed to straighten tipped teeth, or to better relate upper to lower teeth so that the pressure of chewing is less harmful to the remaining teeth.

Since many people destroy their dentitions with extensive bruxing (rubbing one's teeth against each other when no food is present), it is important that the teeth be as evenly distributed and as upright in the arch as possible to reduce tipping forces.

The endodontist (or the dentist himself) frequently has to do root-canal treatment on one or more teeth, either because a nerve is involved already, will be involved after teeth are prepared for crowns, or because one root has to be removed from a tooth in order to save the other two roots.

Initial Preparation

All of this thinking and planning is usually done before the treatment begins. A sequence is worked out so that step by step, you pass through each dental discipline. A typical example would be the periodontist or hygienist seeing you first to clean up your mouth, scale and root plane your teeth, and teach you plaque control. Scaling may be done either with hand instruments or with an ultrasonic scaler. This ultrasonic scaler has a tip which vibrates very rapidly with very fine, short strokes, and helps remove tartar and plaque from the neck of the tooth. At the same time that the tip is vibrating, water emerges from or near the tip and helps remove the debris. Root planing is usually done with fine hand instruments, beneath the gum margin. It smoothes the roots, removing embedded bacterial products and tartar. This phase, called *initial preparation*, could last several weeks to several months, depending on your mouth and your cooperation with home hygiene.

Simultaneously, any hopeless teeth would be extracted by your dentist or an oral surgeon, and teeth requiring root-canal treatment would be treated. Sometimes, root-canal treatment is done following periodontal therapy. Each mouth differs, but in either example, the root canal treatment is completed before the dentist starts crown preparation.

Definitive Periodontal Treatment

After your mouth has been cleaned up, and perhaps after endodontics or orthodontics has also been performed, you are ready for definitive periodontics. This phase will surgically eliminate any periodontal pockets, build up the width of your gum, and perhaps even build up some of the lost bone with bone grafting techniques available today. Some periodontists prefer to do the entire mouth in one sitting. The advantages are several. All bone work, including bone grafting, is more easily accomplished. You only experience surgery once, rather than on several occasions. Lastly, you only have to take antibiotics and pain killers once, so your digestive and eliminative systems are not repeatedly upset. I personally feel that half-mouth or full-mouth surgery, given all the variables, is the least traumatic method when the procedures are done quickly and efficiently. I stress this because the more rapidly any surgical wound is closed, the less pain there generally is for the patient.

If it happens that your periodontist prefers to accomplish his results in quadrants, you might ask him if he would consider doing it in thirds, or as a half mouth. The larger the area, the fewer times you'll have surgery. There are, of course, exceptions, based on your age, general health, anticipated recuperative response, and discomfort threshold. Your periodontist is best suited to weigh all the variables and give you his recommendations. Since it's your mouth, the final recommendations are in keeping with your own preferences, which you should openly state to him. (See Chapter 10, in the section on periodontics, for more detailed discussion.)

When the surgical phase is finished, whether it is full mouth or sectional, and you have become expert at cleaning your teeth by plaque control, you are now ready to return to your dentist or prosthodontist. Usually, it is best to wait about four months after completion of periodontal surgery (and some dentists prefer six months) for the gum to mature before the dentist begins his tooth preparation for crowns.

Many times he will have already begun part of the tooth preparation right after periodontal scaling and root planing, and orthodontics. He has begun tooth reduction (drilling) at that time, but before periodontal surgery, by reducing the size of your teeth with high-speed diamond drills. This is followed by his making a provisional or temporary bridge for you. He does this from casts he has taken of your mouth. The day he does this for you, you go to his office with your current tooth arrangement. He anesthetizes you and works intensively for several hours on a group of teeth, and . . . lo and behold, you have a beautiful, provisional plastic bridge of teeth, which has improved on the size and arrangement of your own, while replacing any missing teeth. This bridge is called provisional because it serves as a transitional or interim bridge until your final bridge can be made. This provisional bridge also helps stabilize any loose teeth, so that during healing from periodontal surgery, the bone can repair most easily.

If you did not have this step early in treatment, you will have it after periodontal therapy is finished. Your dentist's succeeding procedures include taking impressions of your teeth, trying in individual crowns, taking a relationship of each crown to the other within an arch, getting the dental laboratory to solder the crowns together, trying the group of teeth in, and relating the teeth on the lower jaw to the upper jaw. One day, after all steps, you will sit and the dentist will try in the new permanent teeth.

At this point, they are shaped to final satisfaction, the bite checked precisely, and then sent back to the laboratory for final glazing. This produces the lifelike shine that natural teeth have. Your dentist gets the teeth back from the dental laboratory and now tries them in again. If all goes well, you walk out with your permanent teeth temporarily cemented, so you can check their comfort. When you report to him that they feel well, perhaps after a few final bite adjustments, he then cements them in permanently.

All this is a brief description of full-mouth reconstruction. It is very complicated, requires many talents, and a team approach to produce ideal restorative dental treatment—the best plan possible for you. Even if your work has to be done more slowly, over two or three years, to allow you to budget the expense, it is still better for you in the long run to try to follow the ideal treatment plan. If finances just won't permit it, you can still help your mouth a great deal. Here's how. . . .

The Compromise Treatment Plan

When might one consider not going along with the ideal treatment plan? Usually, the reason for not going for the maximum is money. There are not that many people in a financial position to undertake spending $8,000 to $15,000 on their mouths, even over a two- or three-year period. Does that mean that you have to give up if your mouth needs extensive repairs? *No*, not at all! There are other dental approaches, which also may help you keep your teeth. Remember, in all treatment plans, the key steps are to eliminate infection in the gum and bone around teeth that can be saved, and extract hopeless teeth. Now, what variables are left that might be handled differently at lower costs?

Let's take each of the three areas we've already discussed (endodontics, periodontics, and restorative dentistry), and see how we could come up with a lower dental bill for you, by eliminating certain dental work which if done might put the whole plan beyond your financial reach.

ENDODONTICS   The first obvious compromise is to not do the root-canal treatment on a particular tooth unless it is a key tooth. In other words, this key tooth must be saved or the entire dental plan changes. So if a tooth is not a key tooth, extract it. Savings here could be as much as $800, considering costs of root canal, posts, and a crown.

If there are several teeth requiring root canals, then it might be best to extract them, and consider a removable partial denture.

Sometimes, root-canal treatment is recommended to redo old root canals. Here I would suggest that the dentist or endodontist first look at older X rays and see if the questionable area at the root tip is larger now than in past years, since the original root canal was done. If there is no change in size over several years, it might be possible to not redo the root canal, because most likely this is already an arrested infection.

An operation called an *apico-ectomy* can sometimes be done, particularly on an old root canal tooth, which would salvage the tooth. This procedure will be explained in Chapter 9.

PERIODONTICS   Extract any teeth that are too mobile.

Extract any teeth that require bone grafting, should those teeth have a questionable future even if the grafts took.

Extract any molar teeth that have periodontal disease invading the bone surrounding the roots. This is more important on the upper molar. Lower molars seem to hold up somewhat better.

Extract any teeth that are very disruptive to creating a normal occlusion, because they are in poor position spatially in the dental arch.

Extract any teeth that have less than 35 percent bone support and mobility, or have a deep pocket, even on one side, approaching the tip of the root.

By removing teeth falling into the above categories, there would be less periodontal treatment needed, and the final restorative dental plan would be simpler and probably cost less.

RESTORATIVE DENTAL PLAN   By following the suggestions above, there would probably be fewer questionable teeth remaining. Now certain decisions have to be made for the remaining teeth. Would they best be preserved for as long as possible by having fixed or permanent bridgework, or by using a partial denture (a removable appliance)? The key to this question is to not look on the dental replacements as serving to fill the empty spaces of missing teeth, but rather as *preserving* the remaining teeth *while* filling spaces. In most cases, fixed bridgework will do a better job than a removable bridge (partial denture). The reason for this is that most partials are made with clasps, which over a period of time exert a twisting, torquing action on the teeth they surround. This tends to loosen the tooth in the socket, accelerating bone destruction, and frequently leading to loss of the tooth.

There are many ways to design a partial so as to reduce this possibility. One way is to crown and join together two teeth, one of which will be held by the partial clasp. This reduces the torquing force. Another additional method is to use special attachments with slots in the crown of the tooth receiving the partial. The partial itself is built with special extensions. These extensions insert into the crowns on certain key teeth and help reduce the stress on the teeth in addition to giving a better cosmetic appearance. You don't show clasps or hooks. The following photographs illustrate some of the combinations possible with crowns, and removable partial dentures with special attachments.

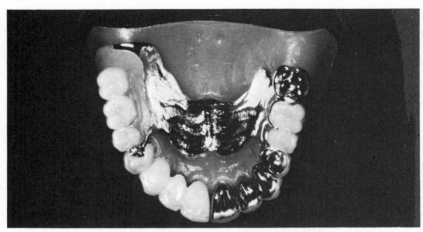

CROWNS AND REMOVABLE PARTIAL BRIDGE

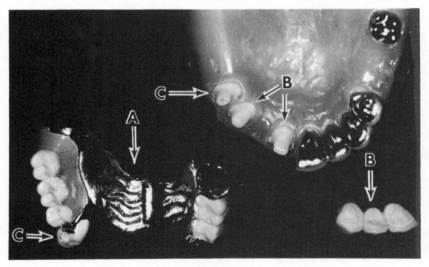

PARTIAL BRIDGE

Still, if it were my mouth, I would try to avoid a partial if I could afford a fixed bridge.

Now, what do you do if your teeth are all somewhat loose and periodontally involved, and you do not want to have many extracted, and can't afford a full rehabilitation?

The solution to this is a combination of conventional dentistry and an approach—used by either periodontists or dentists—called *wire splinting*. The approach to follow here is to have all hopeless or very questionable teeth removed, and then replace all old fillings or decayed teeth with new dental restorations done in amalgam (silver). Teeth requiring crowns in the rear are crowned as needed. Front teeth must all be present in this technique, but a few rear teeth could be missing and the technique still be used.

What the dentist or periodontist now does is drill a groove on the biting surfaces of the rear teeth, to receive a fine, twisted wire or cast metal bar. After placing the wire or bar in the groove, he inserts a white fiberglas-like material called composite into the groove. This sets hard in about ten minutes, and the bite can then be adjusted. The cost of this approach for stabilizing loose teeth is only 25 percent of what it would cost if done by capping and splinting. How long does it hold up? I have seen many wire splints last five years if done with composite under proper tooth preparation principles and isolated from saliva while being done. It is an excellent service where money is a major problem, and if a section breaks, or if one detects decay, this can usually be taken care of easily without redoing the entire splint. Even if the entire splint at some point has to be replaced, since it only cost 25 percent of what caps cost, one could easily replace this splint four times during a fifteen- to twenty-year period if necessary, before equaling the cost of caps.

This type of splint could thus be considered an intermediate restoration. It would allow the dentist or periodontist—and you—to see how well your teeth are holding up following your periodontal care. It would allow you the opportunity of seeing if you could keep your mouth relatively plaque-free. If your dentist thought you were doing well after a few years, if you then wanted to consider capping, it would be with less risk.

What if there are missing rear teeth? Still no problem if there are enough teeth left. It is possible to have a small metal bar (cast in vitallium), which can fit into the grooves drilled by your dentist. Processed onto this bar are one or more plastic teeth to replace the missing ones. As long as there is one strong tooth rear of the missing teeth, and one strong tooth in front, then this intermediate cast-Vitallium splint can be used to stabilize your remaining teeth. It, too, is cemented in with the fiberglas-like material composite.

I have used these for as long as five years. They work well on rear teeth. But if you're missing, or are going to lose, a front tooth, you should have permanent bridgework.

How About the Bare-Essential Treatment Plan?

Here again, one has all hopeless teeth removed. Then, all teeth needing root-canal treatment are removed. All teeth requiring any major periodontal treatment—as already described under the Compromise Treatment Plan—are removed. You now have left only those teeth whose future is predictable. They are definitely worth saving. At this point, you should be taught plaque control, your teeth and roots should be thoroughly cleaned and scaled, all decay should be removed, and either cement or amalgam (silver) restorations should be placed. You now are placed in a holding pattern and should see your dentist every two months for thorough cleaning and scaling, and cavity check. If you have missing teeth, a simple partial should be made, until you are more financially able to consider a better dental plan. Within twelve months, you should try to save enough money, or work out a bank plan, or a time-payment plan with your dentist to at least allow him to proceed to the Compromise Treatment Plan. If you still cannot, then you should go to a dental school, hospital, or clinic. If, however, you can afford more comprehensive treatment after the twelve-month "holding" plan, then you rediscuss your options with your dentist and come up with the best overall plan.

THE DIFFERENT MATERIALS DENTISTS USE IN YOUR MOUTH

Silver Fillings

Silver amalgams are basically used to literally fill the hole drilled by the dentist to eliminate caries that have occurred in the mouth. Caries is the proper name for decay, although frequently we hear the term "cavity" used. Actually, a cavity is just a hole and doesn't really describe the decay of the tooth very well. When a dentist determines that a tooth has decay, he not only drills out the decay but prepares the hole he is making to retain the material he expects to use to fill the hole. Such a prepared hole may be filled with amalgam or, if the hole is prepared differently, then a gold inlay or onlay is inserted into it and cemented in place. Even though your mouth may already have lots of silver in it, it's important for you to understand the difference between silver and gold, and when each is used.

Basically, the difference between a gold inlay or onlay and the silver amalgam has to do with a physical property called *retention*. Amalgam is soft when inserted and later becomes hard. It expands slightly, forcing itself directly against the prepared cavity walls. Its adaptation is better than a gold onlay or inlay, which always has a thin surface of cement between the metal and tooth. But it has a major disadvantage. The amalgam, acting as only a filling, does nothing to strengthen the tooth or prevent it from fracture. The onlay will support the remaining tooth structure.

If a tooth has been filled more than once, or if a new filling would be very large, it may be better to get an onlay, which can actually strengthen the tooth by extending slightly over the cusp edges toward the cheek and tongue, literally grabbing hold of the cusps of the tooth. The onlay, as well as the inlay, has some other advantages. It is carved three-dimensionally on the tooth if it is being done in the mouth, or more frequently on a model at a dental laboratory, and can be better shaped than the silver filling being held by a metal band.

The onlay and inlay can be highly polished and can be better contoured than the silver filling. The high polish will help resist corrosion and pitting, which frequently lead to failure of the silver amalgam. The better contouring is more protective of the gingiva, and may allow food to deflect better while chewing.

The difference between an onlay and an inlay is that the onlay extends over the edge of the cusps on the biting surface, whereas the inlay is retained within the heights of the cusps. The inlay is usually used when the decayed tooth area is small, whereas the onlay is used if the decay has been extensive, or if the tooth has previously been filled.

There are several reasons why your dentist may prefer to recommend a silver filling. The first reason is cost. Inlays or onlays, which are made of gold, may cost between $150 and $300, as compared to a silver filling, which may cost $15 to $75.

The age of a patient may be a factor. For people in their teens, silver fillings will serve well, if done carefully.

Another reason for silver amalgam would be the size of the cavity. If it is small, and especially if it is restricted to the occlusal, or biting surface of the tooth, silver amalgam is perfectly acceptable.

If silver amalgam is recommended, it lasts longest when placed under dry conditions. Ideally, this means under rubber dam, which is a thin sheet of rubber placed over a group of teeth, through which emerges the single tooth to be worked on. Most frequently, however, dentists use cotton rolls to create a dry environment. If your dentist takes the care to use a rubber dam, appreciate him. He deserves it. With good technique, cotton rolls may be successfully used to isolate the tooth, although saliva frequently gets the cotton wet. If the amalgam mixture is kept dry, the filling will be less likely to pit and corrode over the years. Also, if the dentist uses the newer mixtures of mercury and silver, which reduce the total amount of mercury, the filling will be harder.

A very important point is that forty-eight hours or more after the filling is placed, it should be highly polished. This will insure that it lasts much longer than if left unpolished. In the latter state, corrosion and pitting are much more likely to occur.

Silicates and Composites

What other filling materials should you be aware of? How about those white-ones, used to fill your front teeth if cavities have occurred. The two types used are called silicates and composites. Today most dentists have converted to composites. Composites are epoxy resins filled with superfine glass beads or crystalline quartz. The advantages of the better composites are color stability and permanency in not washing out as easily as silicates. Silicates are still occasionally used. Both these materials should have a cement base placed first on the prepared tooth structure to prevent irritation of the pulp.

Neither of these filling materials is considered permanent in the sense that silver or gold fillings are. They also cannot be polished as smooth as the metals, and that means they may accumulate more plaque and irritate the gingiva. It goes back to the old truism that "the best dental filling material is your own undecayed teeth." And, because these materials are not very resistant to abrasion, they should not be used on chewing surfaces (the posterior teeth). They would wear out too rapidly. The materials should only be considered filling materials. They do not strengthen the tooth. One could expect them to last between five and ten years.

Crowns and Bridges

A crown is used when a great deal of tooth structure has been destroyed by decay, a tooth has fractured, or frequently when a tooth has had root-canal treatment (in order to avoid a fracture).

There are basically three kinds of crowns used today: the full-cast gold crown, the veneer gold crown, and the newer porcelain-fused-to-metal crown.

For cosmetic reasons, the crown of choice today is the porcelain fused to metal. It is very lifelike, yet strong. The porcelain may be fused to an inner thimble of gold or to a nonprecious metal alloy. Prior to the development of this type of crown, acrylic-veneer crowns were used, and may still be used by some dentists today. They have the disadvantage of the acrylic (a type of plastic) wearing out too quickly. It is difficult to replace this tooth-colored acrylic once it wears off, and as a result this may shorten the life of the bridge.

The solid-gold crown is usually used on the rearmost teeth where it can't be seen. The porcelain fused to metal is used more anteriorly, where one shows the tooth in smiling.

For anterior teeth, the types of crowns used are called porcelain jackets. They differ from porcelain fused to metal because they contain no inner metal thimble upon which porcelain is baked. Porcelain jackets are 100 percent porcelain and as such are very fragile, but provide the most lifelike cosmetic results. Many movie stars have had good natural teeth jacketed, thinking that their dental problems are now over. In many cases, their problems have just begun, because over the years *gum problems frequently develop where the jackets slip under the gum.*

This is true not only of porcelain jackets, but of any crown, or any dental restoration. The surface that is most gentle to your gum lining is that of your own tooth. If a tooth has to be restored, it is best for the restoration to end, wherever possible, above the gum line. This is why many excellent dentists prefer to have a gold collar show above the gum line, between the gum and the porcelain. They are trying to protect the delicate gum tissue by placing the thin, highly polished surface of the gold next to the gum. If they tried to bring the porcelain under the gum line, they would greatly increase the thickness of the crown beneath the gum, leading to gum irritation and, frequently, to breakdown. In the rear of the mouth, it is best to have a gold collar away from the gum margin. In front, if the smile permits, it would also help to have the gold collar end just short of the gum margin to preserve the health of the gum. Remember, nothing is more gentle and healthy to your gum than your own tooth structure.

Now that you know about crowns (caps) and gum health, what should you know about bridges? First of all, let's describe a bridge. A bridge is a series of crowns, at least one of which is replacing a missing tooth. Here are illustrations of two different types of bridges: On each, the missing tooth is replaced by a crown labeled P, for pontic. The pontic is the false tooth. Now that you're oriented to what a bridge looks like, let's look at an actual mouth. The first group of photographs shows the upper arch of a patient with old dentistry and a missing tooth (A), and the upper arch restored with porcelain fused to metal, including a bridge where the missing tooth was (B). The next photograph shows the front view before (A) and after (B) of the same mouth. The bridge in the first group of photographs is the more conventionally used kind. It shows one or more teeth on each side of the space, connected to each other via crowns which are soldered to each other and to the pontic crown. The bridge functions as an intact unit. Once cemented in, it should remain there for the life of the bridge. The second type of bridge, called a *cantilever,* is not frequently used. It permits one false tooth (the pontic) to hang from the crown next to it. It is illustrated in the second set of photographs.

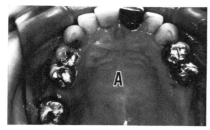

OLD, WORN-OUT DENTISTRY

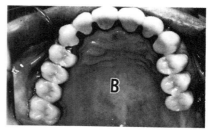

NEW PORCELAIN FUSED TO METAL
CROWNS RESTORES TEETH TO
BETTER HEALTH.

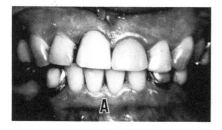

FRONT VIEW OF SAME MOUTH
BEFORE BEING RESTORED

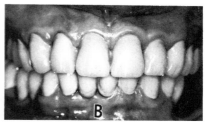

SAME MOUTH WITH NEW
PORCELAIN CROWNS

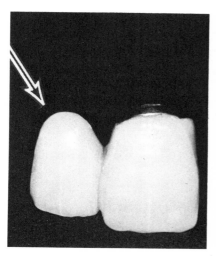

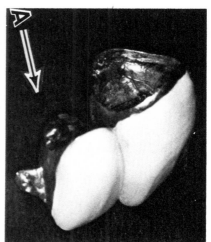

CANTILEVERED BRIDGE. FALSE TOOTH (CROWN) ATTACHED
TO CROWN FITTING ONTO TOOTH.

How long is the life of the bridge, you ask? If a bridge is carefully made, and your hygiene and plaque control is very good, and your intake of sweets very low, you might have a bridge for fifteen to twenty years without any problems.

What problems ultimately arise with a bridge? You might get decay under the bridge after many years. This may require: a) removing the decay and repairing the involved tooth; b) having root canal work done, if the decay gets to the nerve, and then repairing the tooth; c) if the decay is very extensive, the bridge will have to be removed and, after root canal work, a new bridge made; d) periodontal treatment may be needed, with no new dental repair work on the teeth holding the bridge; e) periodontal treatment and steps a, or b, or c may be needed.

Since these problems arise very slowly on a well-made bridge, it is a very useful permanent dental replacement for missing teeth, providing years of use before needing redoing. It is not expected to last your entire life, particularly if placed in your early or middle years, but should last ten to twenty years with good care.

Removable bridges, also called *partial dentures*, are discussed in the chapter on Dental Specialties (Prosthodontics).

In thinking about the length of time any of the above should last, polished silver fillings placed under dry conditions with good bone support could remain a lifetime; the same for well-done inlays or onlays or crowns. Silicates and composites are not considered as permanent as the other materials. Decay can always occur if the dentist makes mechanical errors or if the materials get wet or bloody—and can also occur if the dentist does everything right and you eat sweets, allowing bacteria to produce acids which decay. So if you do get recurrent decay, remember that it may be your own fault if you're not eating correctly or not plaque-controlling.

TEN

The Dental Specialties:
Why Do You Need Them
and When Do You Use Them?

THE DENTAL SPECIALTIES

There are eight specialties that are recognized by the American Dental Association. Of these, six are clinically important for you to be aware of. In addition, there is a discipline: *Implants*, which although not yet a specialty is best discussed as an entity in this section.

The six clinical specialties are:

PEDODONTICS—children's dentistry

PERIODONTICS—treating diseased gum and bone, and helping rebuild the dentally neglected mouth in conjunction with the dentist

PROSTHODONTICS—repairing damaged teeth and mouths and replacing missing teeth and jaw structure

ORAL SURGERY—removing teeth and lesions of the soft and hard tissues of the mouth, repairing fractures, and plastic surgical procedures in the mouth area

ENDODONTICS—root-canal treatment

ORTHODONTICS—straightening teeth, guiding growth and development of the jaws

IMPLANTS (not yet officially a specialty)—placing formed structures onto or into the jawbone to help anchor tooth replacements firmly to the oral tissues.

THE SPECIALIST

What is a specialist? He is a dentist who by virtue of special training, education, and exposure to other more knowledgeable specialists in a particular field, ultimately becomes expert in diagnosing and treating conditions in that field. Frequently this education is a formal two- or three-year training program. It may include special training in a hospital. It usually involves discussing complicated cases. The specialty curriculum tries to cover all known information about problem conditions in that field and ways to solve those problems and return the patient to health. The specialist is trained to set the example in quality care for the rest of his profession in his particular discipline. He actively associates professionally with other specialists in his field, and thus stays very well informed of new developments in his own specialty. He frequently teaches, writes, and tries to share his knowledge with general dentists to inform them of these new developments.

Although some men and women are specialists today by virtue of having helped found that specialty, and having been among the earliest members, most specialists today have had two or three years of extra training beyond dental school to qualify them as specialists. After such a training period, the specialist is called "board eligible." Should he desire to prove his competence further or attain greater peer recognition, he may take an examination given by his own peer group. Passing this examination means that he has met standards of knowledge and care set by his own specialty. He is then "board certified" in his specialty. This does not mean he is any more competent clinically than someone board eligible; it simply means that he has sat before his peers and been acknowledged (certified) as having met their standards.

This degree of education for true specialty recognition must be distinguished from the education of dentists who have taken a course for one day, one week, or one month, or even a sequential one-day-per-week-for-ten-weeks type of course in a specialty. This new training has given the dentist much more familiarity with the particular field, but he still has not had the seasoned benefit—that the specialist gets—of close observation of all types of cases over a period of years. One has to live with one's own failures and his peers' failures as well as successes over a period of time in order to achieve professional maturity in a specialty. There's a school of thought that believes that even a specialist needs three to five years practicing his field before he has sifted out all the information to which he was exposed, tried it, tested it, and seen what works and what doesn't.

In summary, the specialist should represent the highest standards in his field. He is the man to go to when prior treatment has failed, or when you want to avoid future problems if you or your dentist feels that your dental situation is not a simple one.

Let's now look at each of the specialties and become familiar with what the specialist does and how he does it.

PEDODONTICS

This specialty is concerned with the preventing of dental disease in children, and diagnosing and repairing any dental or oral problems that your child might have. Moreover, the pedodontist is specially trained to create a comfortable, non-anxiety-promoting atmosphere for your child, so that he or she may be introduced gently into the world of dentistry. This way the child will not grow up with the fears that so many of the adult population have regarding dental visits.

The pedodontist's primary effort is directed at preventing and arresting decay as early as possible. To help your child maximally, it is necessary for you to know whether your water supply is fluoridated. You must find out how many parts per million (abbreviated ppm) of fluoride are in the water. In conjunction with your pediatrician and/or pedodontist, you find out if any fluoride supplements are needed. If so, they may be recommended either as drops to add to juice or water, or in vitamins. You should establish the need for supplementation *only* with professional advice.

Fluorides taken internally work on the enamel of teeth by forming a harder crystal during tooth development. This crystal is more resistant to decay. Clinical studies have shown that fluoride in the drinking water at optimal levels of 1.0 ppm reduces dental caries in children by 50 percent.

Primary teeth (also called baby or deciduous teeth) begin to form as early as the sixth or eighth week of pregnancy. They begin to calcify *in utero* at five months. Your good diet, balanced with proper protein, dairy, fruits, and vegetables will help the tooth buds form correctly.

At birth, there is active calcification of the primary teeth, and the beginning of calcification of some of the permanent teeth.

After the baby is born, most of his or her early activities relate to the mouth. Breathing, crying, drooling, and nursing are all oral activities. The sucking instinct is most important. The baby obtains nourishment and relieves tension by sucking. Naturally, you might ask whether breast or bottle feeding is better for the baby. This is a highly personal decision, but the prevailing body of knowledge indicates that breast feeding is superior for at least two reasons. The baby's jaw muscles, tongue, and lips are developed more naturally. Secondly, mother's milk is a superior natural product when compared with cow's milk.

If your baby is going to use the bottle, care must be taken in the choice of artificial nipple used. A nipple with holes that are too large may cause fluids to flow too rapidly. The baby, to prevent being drowned, will thrust its tongue against the opening to slow or block the flow of liquid. This can cause a tongue-thrusting habit to develop, which later will lead to abnormal upper- and lower-jaw formation and excessive spacing between the teeth. This is a difficult problem to correct in later years, and frequently requires orthodontic therapy and tongue exercises to correct. Better to avoid the problem in the first place. The Nuk Sauger nipple is well designed for proper feeding and sucking. Ask your pedodontist or pediatrician where to obtain it.

Nursing-Bottle Syndrome

What is "nursing-bottle syndrome," and what harm does it do? You are the cause and your baby is the victim.

Nursing-bottle syndrome refers to a baby having very decayed teeth. The problem occurs most frequently because the parent puts the infant to bed, or even to nap, with a bottle containing milk,

NURSING BOTTLE SYNDROME

juice, or even sugar water or jello water in its mouth. All these liquids have sugar or fermentable carbohydrates in them. The teeth are constantly bathed in the liquids when the nipple is in the mouth. Even if the bottle has fallen to the side, if liquids other than water are still in the mouth, decay can occur. The same can happen even with breast feeding. If the baby is fed and falls asleep on the breast, and is also fed many times throughout the night, the baby's teeth are again exposed to sugar in the form of lactose (milk sugar). The mouth bacteria break the sugar down into acids, decaying the teeth. Usually the upper front teeth decay first, then the upper molars, followed by the lower molars. Last to go are the lower front teeth. This is because the tongue covers the lower teeth while the infant sucks.

Destruction can begin as early as eight to nine months. By age two, most of the primary dentition can be affected. Extensive decay can lead to abscessed teeth, large infections, pain, and early tooth loss.

To reduce the possibility of this extensive decay occurring, feed the baby its milk before placing it in the crib. Then wipe off the teeth with a damp gauze followed by a dry gauze. Put the baby to bed with a plain bottle of water to suck on.

Teething

How can you help your baby when teething begins? There are bacteria in the baby's mouth that accumulate on the gum pads. Starting a few months after birth, simply take a piece of gauze or use the corner of a washcloth to wipe the gum pads once a day. This will remove the plaque, and when the primary teeth erupt they will be entering a cleaner area. As a result, there will be less inflammation associated with teething, and less pain for the baby.

When the teeth are present in the mouth, the same procedure should be used to wipe not only the gums but also those teeth present. When the child is two years old, a soft nylon toothbrush, of small size, can be used instead of gauze. Toothpaste is not necessary.

When should you expect to see the first teeth come in? Generally, at about six months, although there is considerable variation. First the lower front teeth erupt, then the uppers. By the time your child has reached age two and a half, all his primary teeth will probably have erupted.

Baby's First Dental Visit

When should the child first be brought to the dentist? At about age two and a half. The child should then receive his first dental examination. This can be done either by the family dentist or by a pedodontist. You should discuss carefully with your dentist whether or not he enjoys working with children. Your child will sense whether he is caring and patient. Check with your neighbors whether their children have used your dentist. How did they get along? Is part of his office set aside for children? Are there children's books, toys, puzzles, minisize furniture to make children feel comfortable? Are there dental assistants who are friendly toward children? If you feel that your dentist is more oriented to adult dentistry, ask him or your pediatrician to refer you to a pedodontist. Pedodontists (children's dentists) are specially trained to handle all kinds of children, including the difficult ones. They know how to make the child feel comfortable, and how to allay fear. They also know how to sedate, if necessary, and what doses to use for the difficult child. They can help your child start off with good feelings about dentists and dentistry. This is extremely important for the following fifteen years, during which time the child's mouth will either have gotten off to the best start or will have entered the breakdown—fear—avoidance—neglect—more breakdown cycle that so many teenagers experience.

At the time of the child's first examination, he may just be shown around, and introduced to the staff and some of the equipment. Any fear shown by him is fear of the unknown. This fear can be allayed by use of the tell-show-and-do technique. The child is told what will be done. He is shown how it will be done, and then it is done. Successful cooperation occurs because the child takes an active part in the procedure by watching in a small hand mirror what is being done. This eliminates much of the fear of the unknown.

You can help prepare for this visit by eliminating any negative references to dentists or dentistry. Refer to the dentist or pedodontist as your friend, the dentist. Don't say to the child, "the dentist won't hurt you." That's going to make him suspicious and questioning.

Frequently, the pedodontist will wear street clothes, to avoid a clinical look. You and/or your child may be interviewed in a non-dental environment (reception room or consultation room), and a medical and dental history will be taken. The pedodontist can now evaluate the child's behavior, while the child gets used to the new environment. At the conclusion of the interview, the pedodontist will tell the child what will be done that day. Goals should be realistic, and be met. For example: "Now, Billy, we are going to go inside another room and count your teeth, and take some pictures. Then you can go home."

As the parent, you should just give silent support. You may be allowed to accompany your child into the treatment area but you must allow the pedodontist to be the center of the child's attention. If the child is well behaved, he should be lavishly praised. If he exhibits negative behavior, such as crying, he will be told that for you to remain in the room he must stop crying. If he does not, you leave the room, and the child is again told that you will not be permitted to return until the crying stops. When he stops crying, you come back in, the teeth are counted, and pictures taken. The child sees that nothing really bothered him, and he is praised. He may be given a little toy or gift on leaving the office.

The pedodontist is well trained in child psychology. In spite of your protective instincts, for the good of your child, try to let the pedodontist control the situation.

What will the pedodontist be looking for during his exam?

The pedodontist will be checking for any abnormalities of the face, head, neck, glands, lymph nodes, lips, cheeks, tongue, and gums. He will check the bite, and then the teeth.

The pictures he took earlier were X rays. He is going to check for decay, as well as any problems with the permanent teeth buds in the jawbone. He will check for any infection from decayed teeth, and for any fractures. When X rays are taken, your child should always have a lead shield placed over his lap, chest and neck. Thus he will receive no more radiation to the sensitive parts of the body (e.g. reproductive organs) than if he were walking outside for several hours and getting atmospheric radiation from the sky.

The examination and collection of information may also include taking impressions of the mouth for study casts (plaster casts of the teeth). These casts permit diagnosis of potential orthodontic problems.

Finally, the pedodontist will consult with you and tell you what conditions do exist, what caused them, how they can be corrected, and how to prevent future breakdown.

At the second visit, your child will be given oral hygiene instruction, and a cleaning; topical fluoride usually will be applied. These are all easy procedures, and will not alarm the child. On the second or third visit, depending on the child, actual treatment will begin. With the confidence built from the prior two visits, the pedodontist will treat decayed or abscessed teeth as needed. At times, he may be forced to extract a tooth, but will provide an appliance called a space maintainer to replace the lost tooth and prevent shifting of the other teeth, which could lead to a bad bite (malocclusion).

Why Save "Baby Teeth"?

The reason for saving teeth wherever possible is because each tooth is nature's space maintainer. These teeth are needed to help maintain the space for the permanent teeth until they are ready to erupt. Retention of primary teeth until replacement by permanent teeth helps avoid a bad bite.

When children get decay, it can go very rapidly. If the decay reaches the nerve, the child will have pain. We can avoid this by early treatment of decay. If the decay is left untreated, causing a severe infection, the infection may reach deep into the bone and damage the permanent tooth that is forming.

Last, untreated primary teeth can compromise the ideal function and esthetics of the mouth and lower face.

How Does the Pedodontist Treat the Child?

Does he or she get an anesthetic? Yes. Each pedodontist may have a different method of introducing anesthesia, but since he does not want the child to experience pain, a local anesthetic should be used to make the procedure painless. This way, the dental work can be done carefully and thoroughly. All decay is removed and the tooth is rebuilt.

Pedodontists have their own ways of introducing the various materials and equipment to be used. A drill may be called a "tooth washer." Frequently a thin sheet of rubber—called rubber dam—is used to isolate the tooth. This way, the child doesn't even get water in his mouth. He watches in a mirror, and sees the decayed tooth have its decay removed. Then he sees it filled with silver. Finally the rubber dam is removed and the child complimented for his good behavior.

Under the rare circumstances that a child is too uncooperative for the pedodontist, there are some other ways to help the child become a quiet, cooperative patient. The first method involves the use of nitrous oxide (a combination of two gases). This gas can be custom tailored to each child and works very well in relieving anxiety. It can actually make the dental visit pleasant. Young children don't do as well with nitrous oxide as older children, who are better able to understand the explanation of how the gas will help them. The child is not put to sleep with this gas, but simply relaxes.

The second method involves the use of premedication. The child is given either an oral dose or an injection to help put him to sleep. Occasionally, the medication may actually stimulate the child and make him more unmanageable. The pedodontist will carefully evaluate each child before using medication, but he is well trained to decide when it should be used.

The third and last resort employed for a very difficult child is general anesthesia. This technique is resorted to when children are

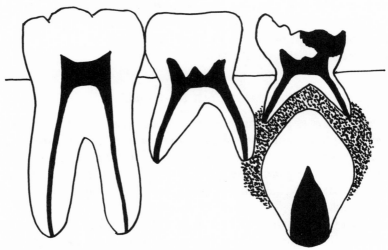

UNTREATED DECAY IN BABY TOOTH WILL CAUSE DAMAGE
TO PERMANENT TOOTH BUD.

under three years of age and need extensive dental treatment. It is
best done in a hospital with trained anesthesiologists. They take all
necessary medical precautions and observe the child carefully before
he is discharged from the hospital.

When Does the Child Go to a Regular Dentist?

The pedodontist will treat your child through the eruption of all
his permanent teeth and well into the teenage years. At that time,
he will suggest that your child is now ready for an adult dentist.

There is another area of major importance in which your pedodontist will help your child. That is the area of *preventive orthodontics*. By preventing the premature loss of primary teeth, either from
decay or accident, he prevents loss of space, which would block out
a permanent tooth or cause drifting and malocclusion in the mixed
dentition (ages six to twelve).

If a tooth is lost in a fall, the pedodontist may use a space maintainer. This piece of metal is placed between teeth to hold the space
open until the permanent tooth grows into proper position. Sometimes a space is too small and a simple appliance can be used to cre-

ate the necessary space. *Space maintainers are most important in the back of the mouth.* In front, space from a missing tooth seems to stay stable without great shifting of adjacent teeth.

Another important situation to be checked by your pedodontist is that of the over-retained tooth. If a primary tooth is retained too long, the permanent tooth may be forced to erupt sideways.

Finally, if habits such as thumbsucking, lip biting, and/or tongue thrusting are present, the pedodontist can help reduce or eliminate them. Failure to do so may result in a malocclusion requiring major orthodontics. Your pedodontist will advise you when and if you should consult an orthodontist.

A final word regarding your children. To make the child's visit pleasant and comfortable, adults must first cope with their own fears and past experiences. A lot of your own fearful feelings, even if you don't verbalize them, come through to your child. If you sincerely feel very negative, and don't think you can easily or positively discuss the desirability of going to the dentist with your child, then you should discuss this with your dentist or pedodontist, to learn what you should say to introduce the subject, and to get the child to go, without prejudicing or frightening him.

PERIODONTICS

Teeth, Gum, and Bone

The field of periodontics concerns itself with the soft and hard tissues that surround your tooth—the gum, the bone, and the periodontal ligament. Your tooth sits in a hole called a socket. It is separated from the socket wall by a thin membrane or ligament composed of millions of fibers plus blood vessels, nerves, lymphatics, and cells. The ligament seems to act as a sling and hydraulic system, preventing the tooth from being overly compressed into the socket. The gum hugs the tooth, like a turtleneck sweater hugs a neck. In health, the gum is attached to the tooth just above the bone crest, where the uppermost portion of the root emerges from the bone. The gum and mucous membrane cover the surface of the bone.

There is a space between healthy gum and tooth. Called a *sulcus,* it is about 1–2 mm deep (⅛ inch). At the bottom of this space, there is a tight adaptation of the gum lining to the tooth enamel. This is called the *epithelial attachment.* Just under this, there are millions of fibers attaching the gum to the root. As you age, the epithelial attachment migrates down the tooth onto the root. It can only do this as the result of slow, chronic periodontal disease. Although your gum space always has some bacteria, as they increase in number they cause your gum lining to ulcerate. At this stage, the space is called a *pocket.* The irritants in the pocket cause a breakdown of the fibers attaching your gum to your tooth. Once the fibers have broken down, the epithelial attachment creeps further down the root, and at an early point, the enzymes and by-products of gum breakdown reach your bone.

What Is Gum and Bone Disease?

When the bacterial irritation and destruction are localized to your gum only, the condition is called *gingivitis.* When it reaches your bone, and the bone begins to be destroyed, it is called *periodontitis.* Gingivitis can frequently be reversed; periodontitis, unfortunately, can only be arrested and treated; the lost bone structure frequently cannot be rebuilt.

The change from normal gums to periodontitis looks like the illustrations on pages 42 and 130. The type of dentist who treats periodontal disease exclusively is called a *periodontist.* His practice is limited to periodontics, which means that he only treats people who have gum and supporting bone problems and/or loose teeth. He has usually had two additional years of training beyond the four-year dental school curriculum, or the equivalent in the clinical practice of periodontics. His background during his specialty training goes deeply into general medicine, oral biology, oral histology, oral bacteriology, immunology, and dental research. Since his discipline deals with both hard and soft tissue, he must be very aware of the life cycle of various cells, especially those of the gum, the bone, and the blood. He must know what happens to these cells when bacteria invade, how the tissue and cells defend, destroy, and adjust, and what would be considered normal versus diseased tissue. His intense focus on these tissues makes him uniquely trained among dentists to recognize the earliest stages of disease of the gum and bone. It also provides him with an early opportunity to treat you and help you prevent loss of more structure.

How Many People Have Periodontal Disease?

Since gum disease (and really, bone disease) is nearly a universal problem, let's look at some statistics. According to one study,* as of age thirteen, 80 percent of a large group of children in the United States already had gum disease. In this study, by age thirty-four, 97 percent of all adults were losing bone. Above the age of thirty, periodontal disease is the greatest single cause of tooth loss. According to the World Health Organization:

> The prevalence and severity of periodontal diseases vary according to geographical, social, local oral, and systemic factors and oral habits. Early signs of periodontal disease are frequently evident by the second decade of life, and advanced destruction is commonly observed after the age of 40 years. WHO data collected from 35 countries show a very high prevalence (over 75%) among persons aged 35–44 years in seven countries, a high prevalence (40–75%) in 13 countries, and a moderate prevalence (less than 40%) in 15 countries. The prevalence in each country was much higher when less advanced stages of the disease were included.
>
> Many surveys have shown the widespread nature of gingivitis in children; a prevalence of over 80% has been reported. The disease is much more prevalent and more severe in many Asian and African countries than in the U.S.A. or Scandinavia.†

* C. D. Marshall-Day, R. G. Stephens, and L. F. Quigley, *Journal of Periodontology* 26:185 (1955).
† "Epidemiology, etiology, and prevention of periodontal diseases," Report of a WHO Scientific Group, Technical Report #621, WHO, Geneva, 1978.

Recognizing Gum Disease

How can you recognize gingivitis (gum) or periodontal disease (disease of tooth-supporting bone)? Why might you need periodontal treatment? Earlier, we listed some telltale signs:

1. Bleeding gums
2. Puffy gums
3. Bad breath
4. Pink toothbrush
5. Enlarged gums with a reddish color
6. Gum recession
7. Spaces between the teeth where no spaces previously existed
8. Loosening teeth
9. Shifting teeth
10. Gum abscesses—puffy, enlarged soreness of the gum
11. Itchiness of the gum
12. Tenderness of the gum

Unfortunately, the disease develops slowly and does not usually cause pain even in the later stages unless an abscess develops. It easily passes from gingivitis to periodontal disease without the patient even being aware. Unlike a toothache, it doesn't let you know that something is wrong. In past decades (and centuries), we just accepted this worsening condition of receding gums and loosening teeth as a normal aging process and assumed that old age meant dentures. This is wrong! We know today that periodontal disease is not inevitable. It can be treated and the teeth saved. We know that gingivitis can be reversed. The key to this is early diagnosis and early treatment. And if you're young enough to still be periodontally healthy, then you can stay that way by removing the cause of early gum disease: bacterial plaque.

The Cause of Gum Disease

The principal cause of gingivitis and periodontal disease is bacterial plaque. We have defined plaque earlier as a sticky, transparent film composed almost entirely of organized bacteria. It also contains small amounts of cells, debris, and saliva. Plaque grows on the tooth above and below the visible gum line. The bacteria in the plaque consist of many different kinds. In a normal mouth, within a shallow gum space, we find mainly round cocci and some non-motile rods. As deeper pockets develop between the gum and the tooth, we find a shift in the bacterial population. Most gum-line bacteria live primarily in the presence of oxygen; deep in the pockets, other bacteria, which live with little or no oxygen, tend to breed. Some of the more harmful bacteria are called *motile rods,* and *spirochetes,* to name a few. Spirochetes and motile rods are associated with more active periodontal disease and bone loss. If periodontal disease is not treated, pockets get deeper as more and more bone is lost. Finally, teeth begin to loosen and abscesses develop. Ultimately, because of more bone loss, and teeth shifting and loosening, the teeth are extracted.

For many years, it was thought that tartar (calculus), which is essentially hardened plaque, caused periodontal disease. Periodontal disease (formerly called pyorrhea) is now known to be caused by the organized bacterial plaque, and tartar is considered an important secondary causative factor. Usually on the surface of the hardened tartar is a living coating of bacteria. Because the tartar's surface is so rough, it may irritate the tissue lining of the gum, in addition to serving as a useful surface for the bacteria to cling to as they organize. *For this reason, it is most important for tartar to be removed at least every three months by a professionally trained person (either a dentist, periodontist, or hygienist). If you keep your teeth extremely clean, you may only need a professional scaling and root planing every six months.*

Since plaque can harden into tartar if not removed within twenty-four to thirty-six hours, it is most important for you to remove your plaque daily. Once it has hardened, you no longer can remove it; the dentist or dental hygienist has to do it for you.

Let's look at the relationship of plaque, tartar, and the gum lining. We see that on top of the hardened tartar (which is adhering to the tooth), we have the living layer of bacteria. It lies directly against the lining epithelial cells of the gum, irritating and ulcerating them.

Because of plaque's importance, I want to repeat the following:

1. Organized plaque is the enemy.

2. After removal, it reforms in twenty-four hours.

3. If not cleaned off, it hardens in thirty-six to forty-eight hours.

4. At that stage, you can no longer remove it, but must go to the dental office.

5. On the surface of the tartar is still more living plaque, destroying your gum and bone.

6. If this process continues, as more bone is lost, teeth get loose, abscess, and must be removed.

Disclosing Plaque

In order for you to see plaque, I described in Chapter 2 the use of disclosing solution. There are several available. Two of the best are the red dye tablets or liquid, and the yellow dye used with the blue light (Plak-Chek).

The disclosing dyes should be used *after* flossing and brushing for maximum effectiveness. That way you can tell if you've really removed the plaque. Examine with a good light. The areas you still see stained are dirty; that's plaque. Clean off the areas near the sides of the teeth where teeth touch each other with floss, and those areas near the gum line on the front or tongue side of the tooth with a brush.

Do this disclosing daily at first until you really know your mouth, and later three times a week. *You really don't know if you've effectively removed the plaque if you don't disclose.* It's like trying to lose weight without checking yourself on a scale or looking in a mirror. You need a guideline; the disclosing solution is it.

Besides your own oral hygiene, and calculus that has not been removed, there are other factors that contribute to plaque retention. These include:

1. Crowded teeth
2. Improperly fitting fillings, crowns, onlays, or inlays
3. Design and presence of a removal bridge
4. A poorly shaped crown, or bridge

5. Breathing through your mouth instead of through your nose, when sleeping

6. Soft diet, with plaque-forming foods

What other factors may contribute to gum disease? Most gum disease is caused by a combination of poor oral hygiene over many years, lack of calculus removal, factors beyond patient control such as quality and design of your dental restorations, and lack of diagnosis and treatment of early gum breakdown. In addition, because of the real difficulty in getting you, the patient, to change your behavior and learn to floss once a day, even the most conscientious dentists have become disenchanted with teaching plaque control in their office. The estimates of how many dental offices in the country are teaching plaque control vary, but the most commonly quoted figures I've heard vary between 5 and 10 percent. That means at most, only 10 percent of the dental offices have a committed, well-run plaque-control program for you. The other 90 percent are still primarily repair oriented. If repair is all you're getting, and since the average filling breaks down in about two years, how can you ever get off the repair-breakdown cycle unless you learn to control your own bacteria? You must find a dentist or hygienist who will work with you and teach you plaque control, and then you must do it, once a day, or . . . realize that you're doomed to continuing breakdown and ever-increasing bills for dental repair. And realize that even with good plaque control, according to the most recent research, many people require professional scaling and root curettage (smoothing) at least every three months to remove new deposits of calculus that form above and below the gum line.

TREATMENT OF GINGIVITIS AND PERIODONTAL DISEASE

Gingivitis

Gingivitis is treated by one or more visits to the dental office for thorough professional scaling and polishing* of the teeth, and perhaps for a procedure called *root planing*. This phase of treatment is frequently called *initial preparation*. It is the first stage of all periodontal treatment, and will allow a clinician to know whether or not you subsequently will require any surgical procedures. In these scaling and root-planing procedures, it is the hard structure of the tooth from which the calculus is being removed. The therapist attempts to get the surface of the root as smooth as possible. This smoothness helps reduce the amount of bacterial plaque that will reorganize on the tooth. Simultaneously, you should be instructed in plaque control, and checked and rechecked until you've got the techniques down pat. It is frequently most beneficial for you actually to be taught and to perform the plaque control first for several days before the professional cleaning, so you can actually see the change in your gum color and consistency. After four or five days, you will be amazed to see bleeding gums stop bleeding, tissues firm up, and redness turn to pink at the gum margin.

As the professional therapist removes any of the hardened deposits, particularly those under the gum or near the gum margin, you will note continuing improvement. At the point where no further change in tissue color or form occurs with additional scaling or root planing, a reevaluation of pocket depth should be made by the dentist or periodontist. Very often, pockets have shrunk from 4 to 2 mm. At that level, the gum space is maintainable by you with plaque control and periodic visits to the dentist. At this point, the dentist or periodontist may remove any "overhanging" metal mar-

---

* The word "cleaning" is a poor term. In some dentists' minds, it means scaling and polishing. To others, it means only polishing. The term "cleaning" should not be used, but when it is, think of it only as a polishing. Scaling would include removal of calculus. It may be done above the gum line only or extend into the gum space. The same is true for root planing, in which fine instruments are also used to remove not only the calculus but imbedded material and softened root structure.

gins near the gum, and polish the fillings that are still usable. This will contribute toward less bacterial collection.

Recognition by your dentist, hygienist, or periodontist of the type of tissue he is dealing with will permit him to determine whether your gum tissue will respond to continued visits of root planing or gum curettage. With younger patients or pregnant women, the tissue is more filled with fluid and will tend to shrink more, reducing the pocket. With many patients above the age of thirty, the degree of shrinkage obtainable from scaling, root planing, and curettage is not enough to reduce the pockets to a manageable level. In these instances, it would be foolish for you as a patient to undergo long, extensive, and costly visits using the above techniques to try to obtain further shrinkage when, in the final analysis, you'll need pocket-elimination surgery. If the remaining pocket depth is greater than 3 mm. (i.e., 4 mm. or deeper) after initial preparation, some surgery is usually needed. A shallow gum space is easier for both you and the dental office to maintain in health over the years. Besides yielding a better result, pocket-elimination surgery can often be done with greater economy of time and cost than curettage. Sometimes, even with 2 or 3 mm. depth in the gum space, a procedure called *gingivoplasty* is needed to thin a heavy gum tissue, thereby making it less food- and plaque-retentive, and easier to keep healthy. This may be done either with a high-speed diamond stone, a surgical instrument, or with electrosurgery.*

Periodontitis

The reason some periodontal surgery is needed when the tissue is firm and the pocket measures 4 mm or beyond is that you cannot clean to the bottom of the gum space with floss, brush, or irrigating salt solutions when the space gets that deep. There are frequently anatomical changes in the root contours at those depths, as well as hidden areas in the root surface that are inaccessible when they are

* Electrosurgery is a technique for removing unwanted gum tissue. The electrosurge utilizes a current. The wire tip can be used to cut or, with various other tips, the electrosurge can be used to stop bleeding (cautery). It is most frequently used to cleanly remove excess gum tissue, to even the gum line, or to provide room in the gum space to permit taking accurate impressions for crowns.

beneath the gum line. These areas harbor and breed bacteria. *A most important study in April 1978 by Waerhaug showed that beyond 3 mm, the most meticulous root planing and curettage failed to leave the tooth surface next to the pocket free of calculus and bacteria. Furthermore, the study showed that the deeper the pocket, the less possible it became to eliminate the harmful plaque and deposits. Only by reducing the depth of the pocket can we make those areas more accessible, and also encourage a change from the more harmful type of bacteria to the less harmful type living in shallower gum spaces.*

MORE FACTS ABOUT PERIODONTICS

There are several logical questions that you may still want answered. What does a dentist or periodontist do when he does periodontal surgery? Will it hurt? What does it cost? How will the results of surgery change the appearance of my mouth? Will my loose teeth get tighter? I have heard my teeth will be sensitive later—is that true? Will I need extensive dental work also? How will I know? How long does treatment take? Will it last? Can I still lose my teeth?

Let's try to answer each of these questions, step by step.

Pre-surgical Preparation

When the periodontist remeasures the pocket and finds the probe goes too deeply (4 mm or more), or finds that there is still some bleeding coming from the base or lining of the pocket, he knows he must treat the diseased gum more completely. He assesses the following:

1. How deep are the remaining pockets? Would more root planing shrink the pocket enough to be manageable, or would a surgical procedure work better?

2. What type of tissue will he be working on (thin, thick, fragile, dense, fibrotic, etc.)?

3. What is the shape, form, thickness, and density of the bone surrounding the tooth? Both clinical examination and X rays yield this information.

4. Does the bone loss extend around the roots? Should any mul-

tirooted teeth receive root-canal treatment so that individual roots which have lost much bone support may be removed at the time of periodontal surgery while still saving the tooth?

5. Are any teeth too loose to undergo periodontal surgery without stabilizing (joining) them? If so, they must be stabilized before periodontal treatment. Stabilization may be accomplished either by using wire or nylon cord placed in a channel or groove the dentist prepares in the teeth, which is then covered with a tooth-colored filling material. Front teeth usually are channeled on the inside or tongue side; rear teeth are channeled on the biting surfaces. Sometimes wire or nylon is wrapped around the teeth, and the wire or nylon may even be covered with tooth-colored material. This method is more bulky and less esthetic. Sometimes, bonding techniques are used.

6. Esthetics: If any of the front teeth are going to be lost, are already lost, or are very loose, then frequently a *provisional splint* must be made. This is an esthetic duplication of the patient's original teeth before the surgical phase of treatment—or actually an improved rendition based on combined discussion between dentist and patient as to what changes the patient would like in his new teeth. A provisional splint is also very helpful for patients who have high liplines when they smile, as the splint will aid their appearance during the healing phases of treatment.

7. Removal of old dental work or preexisting problems. Before entering into the surgical phase of periodontal therapy, any existing infections, such as root-canal abscesses (periapical abscesses) or deep decay, should be removed. Frequently the old dental work, particularly crowns or bridgework, may be too large and would make access to the critically important areas in the gum and bone difficult. Here too it helps to remove the old work first and then put on a provisional crown or bridge before proceeding with periodontal care.

All of the above, and more, go through the periodontist's mind as he plans and anticipates stages in your treatment.

Periodontal Surgery

You have had one or more visits of scaling, root planing, and perhaps gum curettage. You have been taught plaque control. Your mouth is now ready for the next phase. What will it be? And will it hurt?

Although there is frequently controversy among clinicians as to which approach works better, surgery or nonsurgery (curettage) to eliminate pockets, with proper definition of terms there is greater agreement regarding objectives of treatment. Curettage should be described as root curettage, as distinguished from soft-tissue curettage. These are two different procedures. There is general agreement that *root curettage*, or root planing, is essential to obtain a good healthy periodontium. It removes contaminated areas of the root, allowing re-adaptation of healing tissue, and sometimes re-attachment of tissue. *Soft-tissue curettage*, when practiced correctly, is a surgical procedure partially removing the gum lining to shrink pockets. It should be done under local anesthesia; sometimes a periodontal dressing is then placed over the area. Many outstanding periodontists agree that definitive surgery with a scalpel gives a much better-shaped and quicker-healing wound than the less precise soft-tissue curettage approach. When problems involve bone loss and anatomic pathology, many periodontists feel that the moderately diseased periodontium does best with some bone recontouring, and perhaps bone grafting. This seems to best eliminate pockets over a long period of time, other factors being equal. Extremely severe cases seem to do best with a surgical procedure called a *Widman flap*, in which much diseased tissue is removed by direct vision and access, but little or no bone removal is done. Depending on the bone anatomy surrounding teeth, bone grafts may be appropriate to build up lost bone structure. Though not always successful, there have been enough positive results to warrant the use of bone grafts when indicated. These surgical considerations basically sum up the conclusions of a most important recent symposium that focused on appropriate treatment choices for various stages of periodontal disease; and the most recent periodontal literature.

When any of these surgical procedures are followed, a dressing or periodontal pack may be placed over the area treated. This pack looks like a thin rope of pink clay, and is used both to hold the gum against the tooth and to control any leakage of blood. The periodontist or dentist should give you some advice or prescription for any pain that might occur when the anesthesia wears off. Usually, it will be quite minimal, and Tylenol or Bufferin should do the job. If pain is severe, Demerol or Percocet may be used if there is no medical contraindication.

Surgical procedures may be used for different sections of the mouth at different visits, or they may be combined and accomplished all at one visit. Some people, because of age, health, psychological makeup, or too advanced a condition, may not be good candidates for surgical procedures. For them, root curettage at frequent intervals, with perhaps minor flap (gum-trimming) work, may be the only treatment possible. In addition, root curettage and soft-tissue curettage are useful over the years when a great deal of capping has been done to help maintain the gum tissue in health. The better the caps, the less soft-tissue curettage is necessary, as the caps won't irritate the gum, causing tissue to swell. Soft-tissue curettage is thus used mainly to reduce swelling in the gum tissue, whereas root curettage is used to control periodontal disease in a patient before and after pocket elimination or pocket reduction.

What Are the Objectives of Periodontal Therapy?

The periodontist or dentist wants patients to have no deep pockets, just shallow gum spaces that they can easily clean on a daily basis. This means that the anatomy of the gum and bone must be correctly shaped to permit this cleansing. *It also means that any dental restorations (fillings, onlays, bridges, etc.) in the mouth should also permit ease of plaque control, especially flossing.* If they don't, because the patient can't get in between teeth, or the dentistry causes floss to snag, the restoration should be replaced.

One exception to this replacement would be if roots were too close together and the dentistry were well done. Then, other cleaning methods such as a Perio-Aid must be used.

What Types of Periodontal Surgery Are Used Today?

Most periodontal surgery today consists of laying back the gum (like a flap) under local anesthesia. This reveals the underlying root and bone structure, allowing the periodontist to remove the results of past periodontal disease. As the gum is laid back, part of the diseased inner lining of the gum is also removed, leaving a healthy wall of gum. All subgingival calculus still remaining on the root is removed, and the roots are planed smooth to remove deeply embedded bacterial debris. The bone is treated by removing the diseased tissue found at the bone crest, and then the shape of the bone is examined. There are certain anatomic requirements for the healthy bone that the periodontist sculpts and recontours into the damaged bone crest. At times, when too much bone has been lost, the periodontist builds new bone.

Bone grafting is the procedure used to build up missing bone. There are various ways to obtain the donor bone. It may come from within the patient's mouth, from a nearby bony area where the bone is very thick. It may come from other areas in the mouth, such as behind the upper last teeth or even from a healed extraction site. In any event, the periodontist will know, should he elect to bone-graft, which area should be used as a donor site. In addition to this oral source of bone, good results have also been obtained from using other areas of the body for the donor bone. Sterile, freeze-dried marrow bone, obtained by an orthopedic surgeon from the hip, is sometimes used with good results. Other materials have been tried over the years, but the results have ranged from poor to inconsistent, or have been unpredictable.

The success of bone grafting varies, depending on the area chosen, the type of defect into which the graft is placed, the periodontist's technical skills, and certain variables not controllable by the periodontist or patient. For example, teeth that have been exposed to periodontal disease for a long period of time (decades) may have a more contaminated root surface, which prevents the graft from forming a living connection to it. This cannot be determined in advance. Since bone grafts, when correctly done in the properly chosen defect, work in at least 50 percent of cases, they are often well worth trying. Sometimes, even if the defect, after healing, is not totally refilled with bone, it is partially filled and one may then go back later and either regraft or contour the bone. Bone grafting is one of our most exciting and hopeful areas in periodontics.

What Other Methods Exist For Treating Bony Pockets?

Frequently, a bony pocket is found next to teeth that have tipped or drifted. These teeth are out of alignment and are frequently being battered by a traumatic bite. If orthodontic treatment is instituted, these teeth frequently can be uprighted, and in the process the bone surrounding the tooth changes its shape. This may at times reduce or eliminate the need for bone surgery. Most frequently it reduces rather than completely eliminates the preexisting problems. If orthodontics is performed, it may take four months to a couple of years, depending on the complexity of the case. Sometimes the periodontal surgery is done in advance, with less bone work but complete elimination of root calculus and abscess tissue. At other times, the periodontal situation is reevaluated after orthodontics, and periodontal surgery performed on those areas still requiring it.

Combinations of antibiotic therapy (usually tetracycline) may be used for short periods of time, in conjunction with subgingival scaling and root planing. There have been reports (by Dr. Paul Keyes) that using a saturated solution of table salt or baking soda to irrigate the gum spaces is helpful in controlling the harmful bacteria. Usually a water-irrigating device (like the Water-Pik) is used to squirt the solution into the gum space under low pressure. Results from this technique at this point in time are extremely limited and thus far the method has not been widely embraced. Most clinicians feel that each patient has to be treated as an individual, and different mouths may require a combination of therapeutic approaches.*

In European and South American countries, chlorhexidine mouthwashes have been successfully used to prevent plaque formation. In the United States, the Food and Drug Administration has not seen fit thus far to adequately trial-test this important material to see if it could not be made commercially available.

How Long Does Periodontal Treatment Take?

Treatment can take as little as eight weeks, and as long as two years if orthodontics is involved. Most cases average between three and six months.

* Also see Chapter 5, "Why Have Periodontal Surgery?"

How About Pain?

This will vary greatly, depending on many factors. Your own pain threshold (i.e., how you interpret pain) is one of the biggest variables. The operator's skill, neatness, and quickness of opening and closing the wound make a difference. Your periodontal surgical procedures may be done in quadrants or as an entire mouth. Regardless of which approach is used, once you have been given local anesthesia (better known as Novocain or "shots") you will be completely numb and will not feel anything during the procedure. You should expect to use some medication to eliminate any pain that may occur after the anesthesia wears off. Modern medications being what they are, your periodontist or dentist certainly will be able to provide you with a prescription to minimize any discomfort you will have.

In recent years, a small but growing number of periodontists have elected to do all the periodontal surgery in one visit so that you, the patient, will not have to experience surgical procedures repeatedly. Some people have assumed that if all sections of the mouth are done at once, there may be much more pain than from one section. Actually, this is not true. Because those periodontists doing full mouth surgery have perfected efficiencies both in their procedures and in their coordination with their surgical assistants, less time is needed to treat each area. Thus the wound is opened and closed more quickly. There is no sacrifice in the quality of the result, yet there is less post-operative pain than one would expect. It is a surgical truism that the less time a wound is open to the air—and in the mouth, to the saliva and bacteria—the less trauma there is to the tissues. The less trauma, the less pain.

Generally speaking, the larger the area done each time, up to and including the entire mouth being done in one visit, the less cumulative pain you will have, assuming quick closure of the operated area. Remember, once you have any pain, you're going to take medication for it anyway. The fewer the number of procedures done, the less frequently you will be taking pain killers and antibiotics, and eating soft foods while wearing a surgical dressing. Therefore, full-mouth surgery has the advantage of your mouth being completed in one visit with the least amount of total medication taken, in comparison to quadrant surgery. In addition, you don't have to think about having surgery a second time!

There are some advantages to quadrant surgery. There may be less pain, but not always. You can eat more normally on the other side of the mouth. You may lose less time from work on each visit, but by the time your entire mouth is finished, you will have lost more time totally. This is because you probably lose lots of time running back and forth to the dental office when you have the surgical procedures done sectionally. With full mouth surgery there are fewer visits. There may be less swelling from sectional surgery since you'll only swell on one side of your face, but swelling only lasts a few days in either case. In both situations, there may be some slight leakage of blood for several hours.

Given the total variables involved in treating a moderate to severe periodontal condition, I feel that one surgical procedure—or at most two—is better accommodated by most people than the other method of doing the surgery in four or more visits. You have less fear and don't have to worry about having repeated surgeries. Usually, you will be sedated at the dental office, and this will also help to relax you. Only if medical, psychological, or age factors (a slower healing response) weigh heavily would I suggest doing periodontal surgery in small sections. This is a personal preference based on my observations after sixteen years of doing periodontal surgery.

What About Sensitive Teeth After Periodontal Treatment?

It is true that initially you may experience sensitivity to heat and cold if you have roots exposed. This is usually temporary and tends to disappear between four and twelve months after periodontal treatment. Its removal may be facilitated by application of special solutions (stannous or sodium fluoride or other solutions) painted onto the root surface. Your own efforts at home, using Sensodyne toothpaste, also may help desensitize the teeth more rapidly. In addition, a new procedure using *ionto phoresis* has yielded some very dramatic results. Ask your dentist to write to Dentelect Corp., Martinez, Ga., for information regarding the equipment needed to reduce sensitivity. At times, when the teeth are in provisional crowns or bridges, there is some sensitivity at the edge of the plastic crown. The sensitivity may be reduced by recementing the crown or crowns or adding a little extra plastic to cover the sensitive area. Some teeth that are unduly sensitive may for the first time require crowns, and occasionally root-canal treatment, if they cannot be adequately desensitized. Usually this type of tooth has greatly reduced bone support, and will be joined to its neighbors with additional crowns (splinting). Sometimes, an old bridge may have to be redone, but not usually for reasons of sensitivity only. In summation, although sensitivity may occur in some mouths, your periodontist or dentist will be able to solve the problem over a period of a few months. Give him your patience and your cooperation.

Will I Need Extensive Dental Work After Periodontal Treatment?

You may or may not. It will depend on several factors. If you are missing teeth, you will need replacements. *If you are going to have a higher gum line on the front teeth, particularly the upper teeth, there will be some spacing between the roots.* You may want to crown six or eight of the upper teeth, so that your smile and speech look and sound normal. For rear teeth, the decision as to whether or not to crown the teeth will depend on the degree of tooth mobility (periodontally involved teeth usually have some looseness to them). If extensive mobility persists after periodontal therapy, including bite adjustment, you may require gentle orthodontic rearrangement of the teeth to create a less traumatic bite, or you may need permanent splinting with crowns. Frequently careful bite adjustment, in which excess stresses on the teeth are removed by selectively grinding "high" or interfering surfaces, will reduce or eliminate tooth mobility. Slight mobility is acceptable and, if I were given a choice between cutting down and capping my teeth versus having *slight* mobility with a good prognosis, I'd choose slight mobility. Remember, I said *slight.* Your periodontist should make the final decision on splinting, based on his evaluation of your teeth during treatment or at the completion of active treatment.

Frequently, on more complicated cases, several consultations are held with the restorative dentist, the periodontist, and you. At that time, an optimum plan is presented to you that will best protect the remaining teeth and their structures. Based on the professional recommendations and your budget, a course of treatment can be arrived at that will accomplish the most for your mouth and still stay within your financial means.

What Does Periodontal Treatment Cost?

Costs vary depending on the course of treatment and infection. Initial preparation of the mouth (scaling and root curettage) prior to surgery, may range from $200 to $500, depending on how many visits are required and what is being done for you.

Surgical fees vary greatly, depending on the type of surgical procedure, the complexity of the case, medical history, the ease or difficulty in obtaining patient cooperation during the actual procedures, whether bone grafting or soft-tissue grafting is being done, and many other variables.

In 1980, very simple cases may range between $800 and $1,200. With cases that have more bone loss, fees may range between $1,500 to $2,500. Advanced cases requiring orthodontics and/or bone grafting, and mouth reconstruction may cost more than $3,000 for the periodontal work (which may or may not include some orthodontic treatment within the fee).

The most important aspect of the fee is the value you place on retaining your teeth. If you save your teeth with the periodontist's help, then you will have saved a great deal of money also, since missing teeth are much more costly to replace than saving your own. The earlier you are treated, the greater the savings will be.

Assuming That I've Gone Through Periodontal Treatment, Will It Last? Can I Still Lose My Teeth?

Generally speaking, with proper planning on the part of your periodontist, your dentist, and yourself, you should be able to retain all the treated teeth, if your professional team so advises you. Sometimes the condition may be so advanced at the time you present yourself that no assurance can be given that all teeth can be saved. Hopeless teeth may have to be removed. If, however, you are treated early enough, and if you are taught plaque control and do it once daily, you should have a fine result (this assumes that you are in good health, with no diabetes or any other condition, which by itself, or as a result of treating it, weakens the gum or bone). You should also understand that since mouth bacteria are always present, as is saliva with its mineral salts, you may still form calculus, upon which bacteria breed. Therefore, *periodic visits to the periodontist and/or dentist approximately three months apart for professional scaling, root planing and polishing are necessary for the treated patient.* These are called *maintenance visits.* Frequent probing should continue to be done, as a relapse in a specific area may occasionally occur. If it does, by going to your dentist and/or periodontist frequently, he will detect the slightest early breakdown and be able to treat it easily.

Remember, you are the biggest variable. If you don't keep the bacteria away from the necks of the teeth daily, you are again susceptible to breakdown. If you do not see your periodontist or dentist frequently for subgingival root planing, you may have a return of periodontal disease. Do not be discouraged if you find that you just are not disciplined enough to do plaque control daily. Just acknowledge it, tell your periodontist or dentist that you have a problem with always doing it, and ask him if you may come in more frequently for professional scalings. Recent studies in Sweden and this country indicate that very frequent professional scalings will help control the disease even in a mouth that is not adequately maintained by the patient, or that has some shallow pockets. Therefore, there are two solutions to follow-up care. You control plaque once a day and go in less frequently for professional scaling, root planing and reexamination or, if you're not as good as you should be, go in more frequently to see your periodontist or dentist and have your teeth professionally scaled. Based on current knowledge, and with this type of approach, you should retain your teeth for many more years than if you neglect them. Your periodontal therapy, by removing results of past disease and eliminating the breeding places of bacteria, will have given you the opportunity to have your teeth, rather than dentures, in your later years. Your own teeth are much more comfortable than dentures. Your own teeth allow you to chew better, speak better, and give you the psychological comfort of knowing that when you go to sleep at night, part of your mouth (the denture) isn't floating in the glass on the night table!

PROSTHODONTICS

Prosthodontics is defined as "the art of making dental appliances and substitutes such as crowns, bridges, artificial dentures, etc."* Most dentists make the above dental replacements, but certain dentists have had special formalized prosthodontic training for two years beyond dental school. They have studied some of the most difficult problems that a dentist may face in rebuilding a mouth. They have had the opportunity to exchange information and work on very difficult cases under supervised instruction. They have had a standard given to them by their faculty of the highest excellence dentistry can offer. Generally, the combined level of instruction in a graduate program is far more detailed, intense, and perfectionist oriented than at the undergraduate level. When they complete the extra two years, these dentists are called prosthodontists, and they join a very small, select group of specially trained men around the country.

Prosthodontists are frequently referred to as courts of last resort. They may be asked to treat very difficult denture patients, or patients who have great difficulty wearing removable appliances. They may be asked to design a stable replacement in a mouth that has very few teeth left, without rocking loose the remaining teeth. They frequently are involved in a service called *mouth rehabilitation* (as are many well-trained dentists), usually in conjunction with a periodontist. Because of their special emphasis during training on the bite, the proper relationship of the jaws to each other, of the jaws to the temporomandibular joint, of the teeth to each other, and of the muscles of the lips and face to the teeth, they—as well as a dentist who has taken many courses in the above areas—are particularly equipped to handle difficult cases.

If you are a patient contemplating a full-mouth rehabilitation, and trying to choose between a well-trained dentist and a prostho-

* *Dorland's Illustrated Medical Dictionary* (Philadelphia: W. B. Saunders).

dontist, these are some logical questions you might ask. Has the general dentist had sufficient experience in full mouth rehabilitation, and does he feel that he can handle all the variables as well as they should be handled for the patient's sake? How will you know, if the dentist says he can do it, that indeed he can? The only way to solve this problem is to ask the dentist if you might meet and talk with a few patients for whom he has done this kind of work, to see how they look and how comfortably they chew. Perhaps a more important question to ask is which periodontist he would like you to work with. If he says that he can do your periodontal work, I'd be very cautious if your mouth has had a good bit of bone loss. I personally would not feel comfortable unless the dentist has had numerous courses in periodontics, during which he was able to get continuous, supervised clinical instruction and an opportunity to follow up his cases later on to see how they were doing. Periodontal treatment is very complicated, and very few general dentists today can obtain the same results a good periodontist can. Therefore, I recommend that you go to a periodontist on your own, and get an opinion from him on the degree of severity of your condition.

You might also have an independent consultation with a second periodontist, and ask him about the dentist wanting to do the mouth rehabilitation. There are many dentists who have the skill to execute it successfully, and many who don't know their own limitations. Since you may be spending between $6,000 and $15,000 on your mouth before you're finished, you really have an obligation to yourself to be with the right team.

In speaking with capable dentists and prosthodontists, I asked them what was paramount in a successful case. Their answers consistently referred to quality, higher standards, wanting better work from laboratories, sending the work back if it didn't meet their standards, and so on. The diagnosis of what each mouth required was another major point. Someone once said, "Many people hear, but few people listen!" Similarly, many people may "look," but few may really "see." The capable dentist's and prosthodontist's search for nuance and detail, their weighted consideration of all aspects of a case, their ability to know when a problem exists, how to solve it, and which peer to go to should they want to discuss an unusual case, all make for a better final result.

Let's discuss some of the more difficult cases well-trained dentists or prosthodontists are asked to treat.

A patient may have only four teeth left in the upper arch and three left on the bottom. Depending on where those teeth are, and how much bone support is left, several possibilities for treatment arise. In some instances, following periodontal treatment, root canal work might be done on the remaining teeth. Next they would be shortened near to the gum, and a certain type of denture called an *overlay denture* made to fit over them and rest on the gum ridge.

Shortening the teeth helps prevent them from being rocked loose. Preserving them instead of extracting them helps maintain the gum and bone ridge upon which the denture sits. Secondly, they help the denture fit more securely. Sometimes the teeth are even joined with a bar, and the denture is made to clip onto the bar, increasing retention.

Knowledge of physics, engineering, biomechanics, as well as considerable clinical expertise, is necessary to plan treatment for the badly broken-down mouth. The well-trained dentist will discuss with the periodontist what the stresses will be on each tooth, depending on the type of prosthesis that is being considered. Jointly, they decide which of all the different possibilities would best protect the remaining teeth, give the patient the comfort and stability they need, and provide the best esthetic result. These type of cases are among the most challenging and satisfying that a well-trained dentist or prosthodontist, and periodontist can treat because they require so much knowledge and skill, and can help a patient so much.

A few suggestions to help you work well with your dentist or prosthodontist might be in order:

1. *Be patient.* They know that you are going through a difficult time and that your mouth may not be comfortable. Tell them your problems and they'll try to help you. Since your rate of progress is influenced by your rate of healing from different procedures, and by time intervals between various phases of laboratory work, you must be patient and realize that the easier you make it for your dental team, the harder they'll try for you.

2. Don't aim for absolute perfection. Your dentist or prosthodontist will enlist your help and judgment at critical steps. Often, by being very careful in designing the provisional or "temporary" plastic

bridge or splint, many problems can be worked out before proceeding to construction of the final rehabilitation. You will be asked your opinion about your tooth form, the length and position of the teeth with regard to your lips and smile, how your speech is, and preferences regarding the color of the teeth. Be specific in your answers and preferences. Don't say, "It's not quite right, but I can't tell you why." The dentist can only deal with a tangible comment. If you think that the teeth should be longer, or more individualized, tell him exactly that. One of the most frequent errors I have seen in rehabilitations is making the newly crowned teeth look too much like "caps" creating perfect symmetry and/or too white a color. Real teeth are whitish-yellow with elements of grey and perhaps brown. Don't ask for "Chiclets." Don't request that all the teeth be in a perfect row. Bring in photographs, if you have them, of your smile. The more information you can give the dentist, the better he can please you.

3. Let your dentist or prosthodontist know at the beginning whether or not you can afford the ideal restorative treatment plan. If you can't, he will discuss other alternatives. Remember that the alternative is a compromise. You will not be getting all the details that could be obtained for the greater cost. Try to choose the plan that would be the best for you health-wise, and even if it takes you two years to pay it off, it's still your best investment.

4. You should know, in case you're going to be receiving a removable appliance (a removable bridge is usually called a partial denture), that there are basically two kinds. One has clasps (hooks) that embrace your tooth. The better kind has what is called a *male attachment*, or *prong*, which fits into a slot in a crown. This permits better seating of the partial, and less lateral pressure on the supporting teeth. The partial with clasps frequently rocks the tooth it's hooked on to, thereby loosening it.

QUESTION FOR THE PROSTHODONTIST

When Is a Fixed Bridge Preferable to a Removable Partial Denture?

Most dentists today, assuming that you can afford the fee, prefer to make a fixed bridge when possible, because they feel it will preserve the remaining teeth better. Assuming proper care is taken with each step of bridge fabrication, it generally yields a more comfortable and functional replacement. The fee will depend on how many teeth will receive crowns on each side of the missing space, and how many teeth are being replaced.

There are times when there is no choice and you must have a partial denture. Usually this happens when the number of teeth missing is such that there would be too long a span between supporting teeth if a fixed bridge was used.

How Are Fees Figured for Removable vs. Fixed Bridgework?

Fees for a removable partial vary from dentist to dentist depending on the time, judgment, techniques, and knowledge of the practitioner. In general, a well-trained dentist's or prosthodontist's fees are higher, but they may put more time and attention into their work. Finally, the quality of the laboratory work, and customization by the dentist at the chair, are also reflected in the fee. Based on the amount of time spent on impression taking and tooth preparation for clasps vs. time for crown preparation, use of special attachments which must be machined, and many other considerations, the more complex the restoration of the mouth, the more costly. It is not a good idea simply to focus on the cost of one dentist's crown or bridge or partial vs. another's, because you are not just paying for a material product. You are paying for diagnostic knowledge, quality, and high standards vs. possible mass production or elimination of important steps. *As with any masterpiece, every bit of effort and genius that goes into the creation of a work of art is critical. The same is true for quality dental care. You get what you pay for, and you can't get quality at bargain basement prices.*

Is There Any Harm Done in "Cutting My Teeth Down"?

If your teeth are prepared for crowns carefully, with adequate cooling, using water or air and spray, the least irritation to the nerve occurs. There always is some irritation, and sometimes nerves will ultimately die, partly because of the total amount of dental trauma they have experienced. However, when a crown is needed for esthetic reasons, or to support a weakened tooth, it is the best restoration when done correctly. Your dentist will only remove enough tooth structure to allow for the thickness of the crown, replacing the tooth structure removed. Since there is a minimum thickness for materials in order for the crown to be cosmetic, that is the minimum amount of tooth structure that will be removed.

Is There Any Guarantee of a Successful Outcome,
Since I'm Spending So Much Money?

Because of the factors causing mouth breakdown, e.g., bacteria, food, and poor hygiene, it is impossible to guarantee anything, because the dentist can't control the patient's behavior. It is possible to say that *assuming the periodontics, endodontics, and prosthodontics are done well, once the active part of treatment is completed, the success of the case depends on the patient, not the doctors. The dental team repairs breakdown. The patient prevents it.* If you can guarantee your dentist perfect plaque control and dietary habits, he can guarantee you a long-lasting result. He can't guarantee *how* long any more than you know how long you'll live. Just remember, your long-term cooperation is the biggest variable.

ORAL AND MAXILLOFACIAL SURGERY

What does an oral surgeon do? He does not just pull teeth. He deals with the management of diseases, deformities and injuries of the teeth, supporting structures, and the jaws and bones of the face. He is a graduate dentist who has spent a minimum of three additional years in an approved hospital residency program in oral and maxillofacial surgery. In order for him to administer general anesthesia, he must fulfill additional specific requirements.

The oral surgeon helps you in many different ways. For example, he is frequently asked to consult with general practitioners and other specialists in dentistry and medicine about diagnostic problems. These may range from sores and ulcerations to nonhealing areas. The mouth frequently acts as a mirror for other bodily illnesses. For example, certain types of leukemia may first show up in the mouth.

Most oral surgeons also have specific training in general anesthetics. This ability to "put your safely to sleep" allows the surgeon to perform many surgical procedures painlessly and safely in his office. When you know that you are going to be temporarily asleep, your fear of surgery is reduced. Your awareness of any pain associated with the various procedures while they are being performed is also eliminated. In addition, the use of in-office general anesthesia may frequently eliminate the need for a costly, inconvenient hospital stay. The general anesthetic is administered almost painlessly by placing a small needle in a vein in the arm. When the oral surgical procedure is finished, you rest in a special recovery area until you are ready to leave. Sometimes, medications are administered intravenously as sedation rather than as a general anesthetic. You would only have this done when your medical condition requires it, or when you wish to remain conscious but partially sedated. So that the procedure will be pain-free, the sedation and local anesthetic are given at the same time. In those instances where your health or the type of surgery you will receive requires overnight nursing care, the oral surgeon will admit you to a hospital and perform the needed surgery there.

The single most frequent dental situation with which the oral surgeon deals is the extraction. He painlessly removes those teeth which cannot be repaired, or are badly infected. With the help of the intravenous anesthetics, it is usually unnecessary to delay surgery while waiting for antibiotics to reduce the infection. It is better for him to remove your infected tooth as soon as possible so the infection may drain and heal rapidly. Very frequently, the oral surgeon is involved in removing impacted teeth. These teeth have not yet erupted into the mouth. They are covered by bone and soft tissue. These impacted teeth may be blocked from erupting properly by the roots of other teeth, or by the bones of the jaws.

Some teeth will grow in directions that will not permit others to erupt.

Your impacted teeth should be removed for a variety of reasons:
1. Impacted teeth should be removed if they cause the surrounding tissues to remain chronically inflamed or infected. Extraction is better than merely removing the soft tissue from around impacted teeth, because this tissue will usually regrow and the problem will return.
2. Impacted teeth should be removed if their growth puts pressure on other teeth. This pressure may cause shifting or crowding of adjacent teeth, or may cause some erosion of a neighboring root surface. This eroded area may be very difficult for the dentist to repair. In some instances, it may lead to the loss of an adjacent tooth. This possible damage is not worth the risk of leaving impacted teeth in place.
3. Frequently, deep periodontal pockets develop between partly impacted third molars and the second molars in front of them. Bacteria as well as food debris often become entrapped between the impacted tooth and the adjacent tooth. Together they act as an irritant. This causes the loss of supporting bone from adjacent teeth, a situation which will require periodontal treatment, or may lead to the loss of a tooth.
4. Impacted teeth should be removed if they are associated with cysts or other types of growths. A cyst, in simple terms, is a fluid-filled sac. A cyst may develop from the soft-tissue capsule surrounding an impacted tooth. If cysts associated with impacted teeth are not removed, large amounts of jawbone may be lost as the cyst grows and expands. A small percentage of cysts may actually change into other types of pathological entities that are more serious.

Impacted teeth requiring removal should be removed at the earliest possible time. The procedure is easiest for the young patient and the recovery will be shortest and smoothest. It is also suggested that you not wait until the impacted teeth or surrounding tissues become painful. Erosion of an adjacent root, loss of supporting bone, or cystic development may occur with no pain whatsoever. By the time a problem with an impacted tooth causes pain, permanent damage to that area of your jaw may have been done.

When possible, it is an advantage for you to have all impacted teeth requiring removal extracted as one surgical procedure, with a general anesthetic or intravenous sedation. This eliminates your unavoidable anxiety regarding future additional surgery. It is all over at once, and all the tissues will heal at one time. The emotional trauma associated in the past with the removal of impacted teeth should be forgotten. Today, intravenous anesthetics during the surgery, medications to reduce swelling and pain, and meticulous post-operative care all help make you quite comfortable.

PROCEDURES FOR SAVING TEETH

Today there are a number of procedures to save teeth that were previously considered hopeless. Two procedures in particular, apical root fenestration and apicoectomy, will help you keep your teeth for a longer time.

When a tooth is infected and root-canal treatment is being done, it often happens that there may be some pain. This is due to the buildup of pressure from gases and fluids. The oral surgeon can create a window in the bone, allowing for pressure release and thus pain relief. This is then followed by completion of the root-canal therapy. The procedure is called *apical root fenestration.*

When there is an infection or cyst associated with the tooth root after root-canal therapy, it is possible to remove the infected tissue or cyst. The surgeon then seals the end of the root so it cannot leak. This procedure can be done for almost any tooth and is called an apicoectomy with retrograde sealing. Teeth treated in this manner have an excellent prognosis.

Another important service the oral surgeon provides is mouth preparation for dentures. If you are going to wear some type of prosthetic appliance or denture comfortably, it is extremely important that the bones and soft tissues of your mouth be smooth and properly shaped. This permits greater comfort and chewing efficiency. The hard and soft tissues of the mouth are best reshaped and recontoured at the time of tooth extraction. Occasionally it is necessary to further reshape the gum and bone after the teeth have been removed and initial healing has taken place.

BIOPSY

There are many pathological processes occurring in the mouth and jaws which require investigation and sometimes further treatment. These entities may include an abnormal growth of either hard or soft tissues. It may also include an ulceration that does not seem to heal. It is often not possible to make a definitive diagnosis of tissue purely by clinical examination and X rays. The biopsy technique will give an exact diagnosis in most cases. The technique consists of the removal of a small section of the tissue in question. If the area to be investigated is small, then the entire tissue in question may be removed. If the area to be investigated is large, then only a part of it will be removed. A small amount of adjacent normal-appearing tissue is usually removed with the specimen for comparison purposes. The biopsy can be done with a local or general anesthetic, is virtually painless, and very safe.

Once the tissue has been removed, it will be sent to an oral pathologist. This person is specially trained to examine these types of tissues and to give a microscopic diagnosis. The clinical findings plus the microscopic diagnosis determine the course of treatment.

Another situation the oral surgeon treats is that of the cyst. A cyst can develop from almost any type of tissue. A cyst may also be called a tumor. A tumor (or neoplasm) is an abnormal new growth of tissue arising from some part of the body. A tumor may develop from almost any type of tissue. We do not have specific answers as to the cause of each type of growth; however, we do know that chronic irritation or injury to the soft tissues of the mouth can lead to the formation of new growths. Constant lip biting, irritation from sharp teeth, tissue trauma from a poorly fitting denture, or repeated injury from an oral habit such as playing with a pin or clasp in the mouth can cause the growth of a tumor. We know that individuals who drink large quantities of alcohol over a period of time have a higher incidence of oral tumors. We know that cigarette smoking, or heavy pipe smoking, is an important contributing factor to the growth of oral tumors. Smoking and heavy drinking combined are even more likely to be responsible for tumors of the mouth.

A tumor may be any color. It may appear as a lump or actual growth, or as a sore that isn't healing. It may be soft or hard, painful or not painful. There may be associated numbness of the lips, teeth or jaws.

Tumors are classified as benign or malignant. A benign growth is one that grows slowly, pushing whatever is near it out of the way. A benign growth generally does not travel or affect other parts of the body.

A malignant growth is one that grows more rapidly and seriously endangers a person by invading whatever tissues or structures are near it. In addition, a malignant tumor may travel through the lymph or blood streams and cause growths in other parts of the body. Some benign growths may become malignant if not treated.

Tumors or abnormal growths should first be biopsied to determine their exact nature. The oral surgeon will do this painlessly.

The diagnosis will dictate the required treatment. The usual treatment for most growths is their complete removal. Sometimes X-ray therapy or drugs may also be used. The smaller the growth, the simpler the treatment—and also, the more predictable the results.

RECONSTRUCTION AND IMPLANTS

There are cases where the continuity of the jaws, other facial bones, or soft tissue must be restored. The reconstruction may be for aesthetics or function or both. The oral surgeon may use your own natural bone, bone from other parts of the body, such as a hip or rib, as well as other substances like metal or plastic, to restore facial appearance and jaw function.

INFECTIONS

An infection is an invasion of the body by germs such as bacteria, fungi, or viruses. Dental infections are common. They may be very serious. The mouth has many types of bacteria and other organisms that normally co-exist peacefully with you. If the organisms penetrate the tissues of the mouth, an infection may result. Bacteria may enter the body through cuts or sores in the mouth, through the dental pulps of teeth, and through periodontal pockets. If not rapidly treated, the infection may spread into the surrounding bone and soft tissues, taking the path of least resistance. The soft tissues of the face and neck are arranged in separate layers called fascial planes, which facilitate the rapid movement of infections. If an infection remains localized, it is called an abscess; if it travels from its original site of origin and involves other tissues, it is called a cellulitis. Most infections are associated with the formation of pus, which is principally the by-product of bacteria. If you have an infection, you may have pain, swelling, a bitter taste in the mouth, and sometimes swollen lymph glands which act as a second line of defense. You may experience a rise in temperature, along with a general feeling of weakness and loss of appetite.

A dental infection may involve the soft tissues of the mouth, the bones of the face along with the soft tissues, and sometimes the bloodstream as well. The pain and swelling may be minimal, or extremely severe. The swelling may be so severe that the eyes may be swollen shut. You may have a serious dental infection and yet feel well enough to work. Conversely, you may be so ill that you must be quickly hospitalized.

If neglected, disastrous consequences can result from severe dental infection. These infections can seriously involve the bones of the face and linger for long periods of time. Tissue beneath the skin can break down, allowing drainage to penetrate the skin. This can cause scarring and facial disfigurement. Serious dental infections can obstruct breathing, and can reach the brain through various pathways, causing a serious or fatal illness.

The oral surgeon rapidly treats infections occurring about the face and mouth. Treatment consists of prescribing the appropriate antibiotic, culturing the infected fluid to identify the causative organisms, adequately draining the infected area, and prescribing medication for the relief of fever and pain. Once this has been accomplished, the cause of the infection must be eliminated. Treatment is directed at being rapid, efficient, and painless. Again, the use of medications and intravenous anesthesia may be used for sedation and pain control. The better your general state of health, the more rapidly you will recover from a dental infection.

SALIVARY GLAND PROBLEMS

There is a variety of diseases of the salivary glands. The most common problems of the salivary glands are swelling of the glands. This may be caused by salivary stones, other types of obstructions, or diseased glandular tissue. One of the best methods used to investigate diseases of the salivary glands is called a sialogram. A special liquid dye is injected into the gland through its natural opening in the mouth and an X ray taken. The dye, which often is therapeutic for many salivary gland problems, outlines the problem. The surgeon then decides if it is necessary to remove a stone, or even a salivary gland, if it is severely diseased.

TEMPOROMANDIBULAR JOINT PROBLEMS

The temporomandibular joint is associated with a multitude of problems, some physical, some emotional and some a combination of both. The most common problem is called temporomandibular joint dysfunction syndrome, or myofacial pain dysfunction syndrome. Its most characteristic features are pain, and perhaps swelling of the temporomandibular joints. There may be painful muscle spasms, clicking and grinding sounds of the joints. Frequently, there is an improper bite or malocclusion. Often, the problem has an emotional component to it. Those patients who are under increased emotional stress seem to be more prone to temporomandibular-joint problems. The symptoms greatly improve as the emotional stress decreases.

The treatment may involve more than one discipline of the health professions. It will include a thorough examination and special X rays to rule out specific joint disease. To break the spasm, muscle relaxants are often recommended. There frequently is need for bite adjustment, and sometimes an orthopedic treatment appliance to relax and reposition the jaw. Spraying of the face next to the joint with ethyl chloride may be used to break the spasm. Muscle injections may also be used, as well as injection of hydrocortisone, procaine, or other medications directly into the joint. Psychological counseling is frequently of great help to get at the underlying factors causing the tension and stress. With the aid of the above, most cases are resolved. On rare occasions, and only as a last resort, joint surgery may be done to remove part of the joint. This should only be done when all else has failed, and the surgical, medical, and psychiatric team agree that the patient could handle the procedure and any physical limitations which might result.

FRACTURES OF THE FACIAL BONE

If you are in an accident, and have a fracture or dislocation of the facial bones, you will usually see an oral surgeon, whose knowledge of the orofacial region is unsurpassed.

A thorough examination and X rays are indicated when there is a history of facial injury. The prompt treatment of fractures of the facial bones is necessary to avoid facial disfigurement and to preserve the proper function of the jaws.

The treatment varies with the types of injury and the bones involved. In general, the fractured bones must be put into their correct alignment (reduced), and fixed (set) in place. This may require wiring the teeth together, which will act as a splint, or sometimes directly wiring the fractured bones together and fixing them in place. Most facial fractures require six to eight weeks to heal.

Orthognathic Surgery (A Special Field)

Developmental facial deformities are deformities which occurred before birth or developed during the early years of the child. Acquired facial deformities occur not as a result of development, but from injuries or habit. Orthognathic surgery is the surgical and orthodontic correction of deformities of the facial bones. During orthognathic surgery, teeth and bones are moved into their correct relationships to achieve a pleasant facial appearance and properly functioning jaws.

For the last twenty-five years in the United States, the oral surgeon has concentrated his research efforts on the correction of facial deformities. Today, almost any type of correction is possible. It is no longer necessary for any person to go through life unable to bring his lips together, or to suffer with a jaw that does not function correctly. Nor does any person have to go through life with an underdeveloped jaw or no chin or, conversely, a jaw that is too large for the rest of his face. These problems have solutions.

The jaws, or sections of jaws, can be moved forward, backward, up and down, or rotated. Teeth in their bony attachments may be moved into many positions. The chin can be moved into different positions and clefts, and other deformities can be corrected. The entire facial structure can be reoriented so that the jaws function properly and the face is esthetically pleasing.

Almost every procedure can be performed from inside the mouth, thus eliminating the problem of facial scarring. Some procedures can be performed in the office, but most orthognathic surgery requires a short hospital stay. The patient is able to function satisfactorily and comfortably during the post-operative healing period.

The correction of facial deformities requires much planning and close cooperation among all dental disciplines. For certain complex problems, like a cleft palate, the team may consist of an oral or plastic surgeon, an orthodontist, a prosthodontist, a pedodontist, and sometimes an ear, nose, and throat specialist. Later, with cleft-palate repair, and depending on the child's age, a pediatrician or a child psychologist, as well as a speech therapist, may be needed. Cleft lip should be treated in the first six months of life, whereas cleft palate can be treated in the second year. There are centers for cleft-palated patients, which will be of help in guiding you.

Tongue-tie is another developmental defect that is easily treated. The operation is very simple, and can be done as early as in a one-week-old infant, or, later on in childhood when speech problems are noticed. The excess tissue holding the tongue is anesthetized and easily removed.

Corrections for most problems can be made at any age. Generally it is suggested that these various surgical corrections be made at an early age, if possible. There will be less psychological scarring, and this may be the most important benefit of all.

THE ENDODONTIST

For many centuries, men have struggled to relieve tooth pain without losing the offending tooth.

Root-canal therapy (endodontics) is one such technique that your dentist or endodontist (a specialist in root-canal problems) can use to save teeth that would otherwise have to be removed due to advanced dental disease.

As we discussed earlier (in Chapter 1), the tooth can be divided into two parts (Fig. 1): the crown and the roots. The number of roots will vary from tooth to tooth, depending on the position of the tooth in the dental arch. The hard tooth has a hollow core. In a healthy tooth, this hollow space contains blood vessels, nerves, and tissue, and these elements collectively are called the *pulp*. The hollow space may be divided into two sections. The space located in the crown of the tooth is known as the *pulp chamber*. The second section, which extends through the roots, is known as the *root canal*. The illustration shows different adult teeth with one or more roots and the corresponding root canals.

The tooth has two sources of blood supply, one inside the tooth, supplying the pulp; and the other outside the tooth, supplying the cementum and periodontal ligament.

When the pulp becoms diseased or injured to such an extent that the tooth can no longer repair itself, root-canal therapy is necessary.

The causes of pulp disease are many and varied, and can be arranged into several groups. Under physical causes, we have trauma without fracture, such as a blow or a fall. This type of accident can

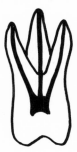 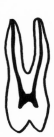 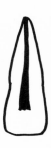 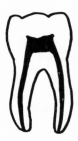

CROSS-SECTION OF ADULT TEETH AND ROOT SYSTEM

interfere with the blood supply to the pulp, and may lead to pulpal death requiring root-canal therapy. Fracture of the tooth exposing the pulp will require treatment. Sometimes a crack in the tooth or a fracture extending only into dentine, if left unattended long enough, will require endodontic treatment.

Heat from drilling teeth, setting of cement, or even polishing of fillings can, at times, be so excessive that pulpal death ensues, and root-canal therapy is necessary.

However, by far the most common cause of pulpal disease is dental decay. Toxins produced by the decay-causing bacteria, or direct invasion of the pulp by these bacteria, may lead to pulpal death.

Dead pulp tissue provides an excellent food source for bacteria. The bacteria multiply and an infection becomes established in the tooth. Eventually, if left untreated, the infection will spread throughout the tooth, then into the periodontal ligament, and then into the jawbone. The infection may continue to spread to the soft tissues of the face, and facial swelling may now be noticed. Even at this late stage, the infection may still be cured and the tooth saved.

As the tooth decays, different signs and symptoms will alert you to what is happening. When decay is still limited to dentine, you may notice sensitivity to sweets, hot, or cold. However, the pain you feel from these stimuli will cease as soon as the stimuli are removed. As the carious process approaches and enters the pulp, you notice that the pain associated with hot and cold will now linger for several seconds or even minutes after the stimulus is removed. When more of the pulp tissue is involved, you notice the beginning of a neuralgic type of pain. This pain cannot usually be localized to a specific tooth and, sometimes may even be referred to different areas in the face. For example, the ear, the eye, or the opposite jaw of the patient may hurt. You may even experience headaches. As the infection approaches the peri-

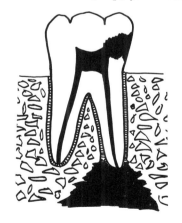

A TOOTH WHICH WILL REQUIRE ROOT CANAL WORK

odontal ligament, at the root tip, a sensitivity to bite pressure develops. Then, as the infection travels in the jawbone, there may be a dramatic reduction of symptoms for a while. Once the infection reaches the soft tissues of the face, painful symptoms will appear and facial swelling may become evident.

During the course of pulpal disease, there may be no symptoms. This can occur when the infection is of a low-grade chronic type. Your dentist may realize that there is pulpal disease only when bone destruction is noticed on routine X rays. On the other hand, the symptoms can be of such severity at any time that they drive the patient to seek professional help immediately.

The actual therapy consists basically of two steps: Initially, the pulp is removed and the root canal is sterilized; then the filling is placed that will replace the lost pulp tissue.

To begin treatment, your dentist or endodontist will probably give you a local anesthetic so that you will feel no discomfort. Next, he will place a sheet of rubber, which has a hole punched in it and which is stretched over a frame, onto your tooth. This "rubber dam" isolates the tooth to be treated from the rest of your mouth and keeps saliva and other contaminants out of the root-canal system.

The dentist, using the high-speed drill, then makes a small opening through the crown of the tooth into the pulp chamber. He inserts endodontic instruments into the root canals. These instruments are used to file and ream the canals clean. At this point, with the endodontic instruments in the tooth, an X ray is taken to determine the exact length of the roots. When the dentist knows this

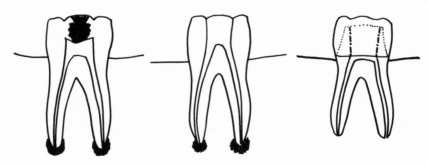

TREATMENT OF PULPAL DISEASE

length, he can be assured only of cleaning out the root canal, not the jawbone beyond the canal. After the root canals have been preliminarily cleaned (using a combination of endodontic instruments and irrigation solution), the dentist places a cotton pellet into the pulp chamber. This pellet has been dipped in a medication whose vapors sterilize the canals. Finally, the opening originally made to enter the pulp chamber is sealed with a temporary cement.

In some cases, if the infection is severe and pus is draining from the tooth, the opening is left unsealed for several days and antibiotics may be given. In other cases, the infection may have passed beyond the tooth and bone and into the soft tissue of the face or neck. If conditions are right, your dentist may incise or lance the swelling inside the mouth, removing the accumulated pus immediately from the tissues, thus accelerating healing. Once the infection is no longer acute, the incision will heal in several days.

The next visit, from your point of view, seems to be about the same as the first visit. Actually, the dentist is cleaning the canals more thoroughly and shaping them to receive the root-canal fillings.

After each visit, you will feel either absolutely fine or experience a small amount of discomfort lasting for one or two days. This soreness is due to inflammation in the periodontal ligament at the root tip created by working on the tooth.

Up until recently, most dentists were using silver points and cement to fill the root canals. However, dental research has now shown that over a long period of time, in some people, the silver tends to corrode. This corrosion leads to inflammation, which in turn leads to infection. Therefore, there has been a general shift from silver to gutta-percha. Gutta-percha is a rubberlike substance that remains relatively inert in the body. The gutta-percha is generally cemented into the canal with one of several types of dental cement. It is then condensed to fill any voids present in the root canal. The object is to create a hermetic seal at the tip of the root canal.

After the root canal is filled, the small opening made in the crown can be restored permanently with a silver or plastic filling, a gold inlay, onlay, or even a porcelain or gold crown. The restoration will depend upon the amount of tooth structure left and the tooth's position in the mouth. If the entire crown of the tooth has broken down, it is possible to build up this missing tooth structure with posts that anchor into the roots and give support to a new crown. Fabrication of post-crowns is a very common procedure.

Dental research shows that the type of endodontic treatment that I have been discussing is successful in ninety to ninety-five cases out of a hundred. However, in that small percentage of cases that are unsuccessful, an alternative form of treatment does exist. It is a surgical procedure using local anesthesia, done in the dental office, and takes only about an hour to complete.

The surgery involves making one or more incisions in the gum tissue and raising a flap of tissue to expose the underlying bone and tooth structure. At this point, several variations in the clinical procedure can take place. Most commonly, the infection is cleaned out, a small portion of the root at its tip is removed, and a silver filling is placed into the root canal at the tip to seal it. The flap of tissue is then sutured back into place. The patient is asked to return in five to seven days to remove the sutures. There is usually slight swelling that lasts for several days and some soreness associated with this procedure. The technical name for this operation is an "apicoectomy with retrograde amalgam." Apicoectomy means removal of the apex of the root, and retrograde amalgam is the placement of the silver filling at the tip of the root. The prognosis for retaining a tooth using this technique is excellent.

Frequently, prior to having a root canal done, a patient asks, "Won't my tooth turn black?" Occasionally, you see somebody with a dark tooth. The causes of tooth discoloration are the same regardless of whether they occur before or after endodontic treatment. The most prevalent cause is the rupture of blood vessels, allowing blood into the pulp chamber. Blood-breakdown products stain the tooth. Debris, if not cleaned out properly during root-canal therapy, also gives rise to tooth-staining compounds. This is one of the reasons dentists take extra care in removing all tissue debris from the canals and pulp chamber.

If staining does occur, *bleaching* can be used to correct the discoloration. The prognosis for correcting the discoloration depends on the cause and type of discoloration present. Usually, staining caused by blood-breakdown products or dead tissue has a good prognosis for removal. On the other hand, discoloration caused by filling materials like silver amalgam or various cements is difficult to bleach satisfactorily.

The bleaching procedure is done after root-canal therapy is completed. The tooth is again isolated by means of the rubber dam, and entered. A mixture of 30 percent hydrogen peroxide and sodium perborate is placed into the pulp chamber. Using a special *procedure*, and a special light, the tooth is effectively bleached. This *procedure* is repeated several times during the visit. The tooth is then closed off, with peroxide and sodium perborate being sealed inside. The mixture remains there until the next visit, which is usually in a week. At this visit, the same *procedure* is repeated until the tooth is slightly lighter than its adjacent tooth. The tooth is then sealed with a permanent filling. The tooth will soon darken slightly, and match the adjacent tooth.

Endodontics today, because of the vast improvement in our knowledge of the disease process and technical skills, can be performed successfully on just about any tooth. There are, however, two instances where endodontics cannot save the tooth.

Fracture of a tooth in a vertical direction cannot be treated with any great success at this time, and therefore extraction is recommended. Also, if a tooth is unrestorable due to extensive decay extending too far below the crest of the jawbone, root-canal therapy should not be done. Since the tooth is unrestorable, it cannot function in a useful manner and it would be foolish to attempt to save such a tooth.

Endodontics, meaning inside the tooth, is a treatment which in the vast majority of cases will enable you to retain an infected tooth that othewise might have to be extracted. Keeping the tooth is not only the best thing for your oral health, but it is also cheaper than extracting it and replacing it with an artificial one.

ORTHODONTICS FOR CHILDREN AND ADULTS

Orthodontics is the science of correcting or straightening teeth; and where possible, guiding the growth and development of the jaws and facial skeleton. The purpose of orthodontics is to provide good looks and properly functioning teeth. When a dentist says that someone has a good bite, or a bad bite, he refers to how the upper and lower teeth come together. Dracula might define a "good bite" differently, but this is, after all, a dental book.

When teeth meet they can be crowded, tipped, or rotated. Those conditions may cause problems. Teeth properly arranged permit ease of chewing, biting,and swallowing.

You can think of the baby teeth as the foundation for the permanent teeth. If the baby teeth come in well, do not decay extensively, and are not lost prematurely, then a good foundation has been prepared for the arrival of the permanent teeth. Behind the last of the baby molars, the six-year molar (the first permanent tooth) comes in. How the upper six-year molar relates to the lower six-year molar will have great bearing on how the final adult bite shapes up. *The period from six to 13 years is called the mixed dentition years. The early years of this period are the best time to guide and plan for any orthodontic assistance to natural growth and development.* During this period, careful observation will head off any future trouble. (See the Eruption Table on page 64.)

After the age of six, through proper X rays and measurements of study casts taken of your child's mouth, it is possible to anticipate potential problems. One can project how the permanent teeth will erupt into the mouth. The dentist is able to measure distances between the teeth on the study casts he has taken of the child's mouth, and decide whether there will be adequate room for all the incoming teeth. If he decides that there will not be enough room, he may recommend interceptive orthodontics. To make a diagnosis, the orthodontist, dentist, or periodontist must analyze tooth-to-jaw relationships, jaw-to-jaw relationships, jaw-to-skull relationships, and soft-tissue relationships (lips, chin, nose, etc.). The orthodontist is concerned particularly with proper growth of the child's jaws and preventing serious facial deformities. He may also correct malrelationships due to various causes with the appropriate treatment. He may treat thumbsucking, correct a crossbite, or maintain space where a tooth has been prematurely lost.

By asking questions of your dentist or pedodontist as the child grows, you will be best able to guide your child to an orthodontist at the right time. This will help your child get off to a good start es-

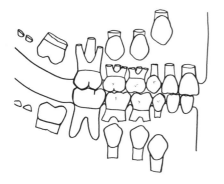

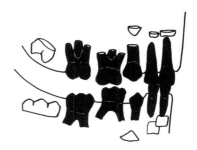

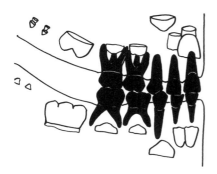

1. ERUPTION OF FIRST SET OF TEETH INTO MOUTH (BABY TEETH). CROWNS OF ADULT TEETH ARE FORMING WITHIN THE JAW

2. BABY TEETH FULLY IN POSITION. CROWNS OF ADULT TEETH ARE DEVELOPING WITHIN JAW.

3. MIXED DENTION, 9 YEARS

thetically and dentally. It may take several years of treatment, but it's one of the best investments in your child's well-being.

Malocclusion is often spoken about in relation to orthodontic care. Let us examine what malocclusion is in order to understand what's done abut it. Malocclusion means an improper meeting of the teeth. To simplify treatment, Dr. Edward Angle, in the 1880s, developed a classification to describe the main types of malocclusion. It is based on the relationship of the upper to the lower teeth, of teeth to one another, the jaw-to-jaw relationship, and the relationship within a jaw. The three basic types are Angle Class I, Class II, and Class III.

Angle's key to the classification is the relationship of the upper first molar to the lower first molar. When the upper and lower teeth fit correctly, the teeth (especially the first molar) appear as in the il-

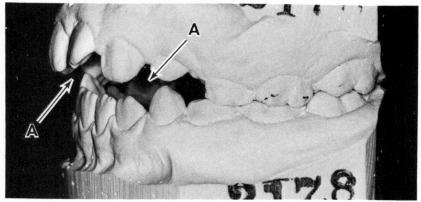

ANGLE CLASS I, WITH OPEN BITE

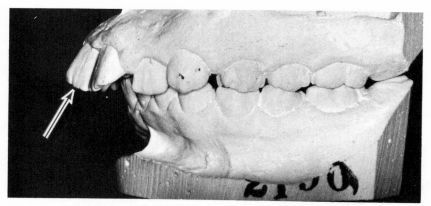

ANGLE CLASS II, WITH SEVERE OVERJET AND OVERBITE

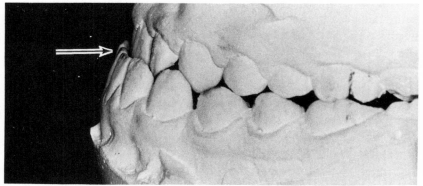

ANGLE CLASS III

lustration for Angle Class I. Even in Class I, which is a correct upper-to-lower-first-molar relationship, individual teeth may still be tipped, crowded, malrotated, or missing.

A Class II malocclusion is the kind you most frequently think of as needing treatment by the orthodontist. This is the "buck tooth" case, where the upper front teeth hang out over the lower, and the lower jaw looks small while the lower teeth bite way behind the uppers, perhaps even hitting the palatal tissue behind the upper front teeth. Here the upper molar is more forward of the lower molar.

A Class III malocclusion is the opposite of a Class II. Here the lower jaw sticks out too much (the phrase "lantern jaw" comes to mind). Lower front teeth are in front of the upper front teeth and when the jaws are closed, the lower first molar is now forward of the upper first molar.

Some other important terms are *overbite, crossbite, deep bite,* and *open bite.*

An *overbite* is the degree to which the upper teeth extend over the lower teeth. The upper front teeth normally extend downward over the lower ones. The vertical distance between the edge of each of the upper and lower incisors would be the degree of overbite, usually measured in millimeters. Similarly, the outer cusps of the

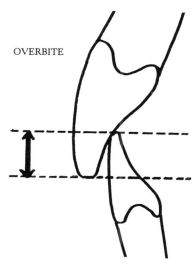

OVERBITE

posterior upper teeth, when in proper relationship with the lower cusps, extend over them.

In *crossbite*, the normal relationship is reversed. Here the lower teeth are outside the uppers when the jaw is closed. It may occur on one side, or both sides of the mouth, or on the front teeth.

A *deep bite* is one in which the upper front teeth cover the lower front teeth so that when you look at the mouth, the lower teeth are hidden.

Open bite. In this condition, two or more teeth in the upper and lower jaw do not make contact when the other teeth are closed. As a result, the teeth cannot completely meet, and the patient has an open bite. An open bite can also be caused by a tongue thrust, in which pressure from the tongue, each time the patient swallows, prevents upper, or upper and lower teeth, from erupting into contact.

Now that we've discussed the basic classification, and some commonly described situations, let's see how these malocclusions developed.

There are many causes of malocclusion. Among them are:

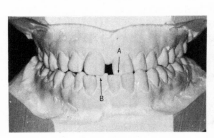

CROSSBITE

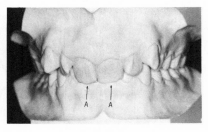

DEEP BITE

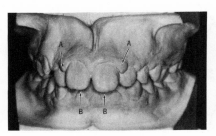

DEEP BITE

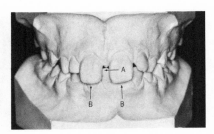

OPEN BITE

1. Early loss of baby teeth due to infection or decay, or a fall. By not filling the space that results from tooth loss with a space maintainer, teeth behind the space drift forward and block the permanent teeth from coming in when they are ready to erupt.

2. Overretention of baby teeth. This blocks out the permanent tooth fighting to erupt under the baby tooth. It prevents the teeth from meeting in a proper manner. This may disturb normal chewing patterns.

3. Tooth size. Teeth that are too small may permit drifting and incorrect arrangement of adjacent teeth. In turn, this may prevent teeth in one arch from meshing well with teeth in the opposite arch. Conversely, teeth that are too large for an arch will lead to crowding. This will cause cusp tips to be misplaced, and may lead to locked bites or slips in chewing which should not occur.

4. Arch size. One could have crowding or spacing not due to tooth size, but to normally sized teeth erupting into an arch that is too big or too small to accommodate them in proper order.

5. Loss or absence of a permanent tooth. If a tooth is lost due to extensive decay and infection, from trauma, or an accident requiring extraction, the tooth should be replaced by a space maintainer or a bridge, or the space closed by moving the remaining teeth into the space. Failure to do this frequently results in a shifting of adjacent teeth on each side of the space, while the opposing tooth extrudes into the space. This disturbs the normal arrangement of the teeth in that area. As teeth tip into the open area, they set up the potential for periodontal breakdown. Tipped teeth receive incorrect pressure when biting, which tends to tip them more. They also tend to collect food debris more easily, which will support bacterial plaque growth.

6. Spacing of front teeth. There may be several causes. They include:

a. A heavy band of tissue (called a *frenum*) inserting between the front teeth frequently causes spacing.

b. An extra, or *supernumerary tooth,* either erupting between the crowns of the two incisors or lodged between the roots, can keep the teeth apart. X rays will help diagnose this possibility.

c. The teeth may be too small for the size of the arch, or the arch may be too big for the size of the tooth.

d. A habit, such as a reverse swallow or tongue thrust, applying pressure to the inside of the upper front teeth, is enough to spread them and keep them spread. Another habit is that of catching the lower lip under the upper teeth. This creates enough pressure to push the uppers out, spreading them.

e. A periodontal pocket in an adult can create enough pressure due to the inflamed tissue to force a front tooth out or make two teeth separate.

f. Again, in the periodontal patient, if there has been loss of the lower six-year molars, or other teeth, the lower jaw in closing frequently slides forward before reaching final maximum tooth closure. This puts pressure on the upper teeth and causes them to spread. The phrase, "teeth taking a walk," refers to this spreading of teeth which did not exist earlier in life.

g. The medical condition called *acromegaly*, or *adult hyperpituitarism*, can cause spreading where none existed.

h. Overgrowth of heavy gum tissue, as in treatment of epilepsy with Dilantin, can be forceful enough to cause spacing.

7. Dental decay on the side of a tooth adjacent to another tooth, causing loss of tooth structure between the teeth. If the rear teeth then drift forward, there can be a loss of space. Subtle, but important, slipping of the bite may then occur, leading to extra pressure on the teeth, or occasionally to pressure in the jaw joint. Any malocclusion may lead to the above sequence of events. Even if teeth are filled, or restored, if not done correctly, there can be a reduction of space between teeth as teeth drift together, because they were not restored to touch each other.

8. Improper muscle balance, weak lips, too powerful a tongue, too powerful a chin muscle, and other imbalances that will put pressure on teeth. Since final tooth position is very much a function of proper balance between many groups of muscles, any imbalances, damage, scarring, paralysis of a nerve supplying the muscle, or over-development of one group of muscles in relationship to another can cause asymmetry of the tooth arrangement.

9. Infections or growths (tumors or cysts) within the jawbone, which can cause a malocclusion to develop, as teeth are pushed to one side. X rays will help reveal this as a causative factor.

10. Noneruption of a permanent tooth. A tooth can be fused to the

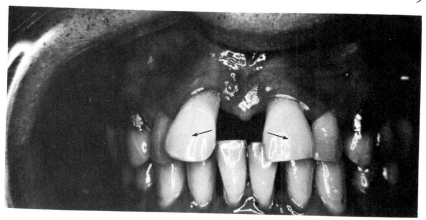

TEETH "TAKING A WALK"

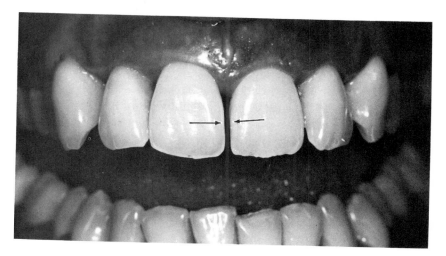

bone surrounding it and fail to erupt. This is called ankylosis. The tooth can also erupt partly and then become ankylosed. In either case, there will be drifting and shifting of adjacent teeth, leading to a malocclusion.

11. Genetic influences: Large jaws, small jaws, extra or missing teeth, tooth size, etc., may run in the family. Although a child represents both sides genetically, there are all sorts of possibilities, de-

pending on which genes are dominant. Here one simply has to recognize early and correct early as needed.

Other factors which might influence jaw relationships and tooth relationships are:

> 1. Mother's diet during pregnancy when jaws and tooth buds are forming
> 2. After birth, nutritional deficiency in the growing baby
> 3. Disease of childhood if very severe (scarlet fever, chicken pox, measles, poliomyelitis)
> 4. Hormonal imbalance, especially the pituitary, thyroid, and parathyroid glands
> 5. Respiratory abnormalities
> 6. Allergies

Now that you understand how malocclusions may occur, it would be good to examine your mouth and your children's mouth.

To examine your child's mouth and determine if they need orthodontics, here are some suggestions:

1. Ask the child to bite closed on his back teeth.

2. Have him place the index and middle fingers of each hand in the corner of his mouth, two on the left and two on the right. Now ask him to push one finger against the upper lip and another downward against the lower lip.

3. Now study the front teeth. Are they apart? Are they tipped, rotated, or overlapped? Can you see the lowers, or are they hidden? Are they crowded? Are the upper and lower front teeth open when the back teeth are closed?

4. Look at the child from the side. Do the upper teeth extend far over the lower?

5. Now take a small teaspoon and, in a good light, with the child's mouth open, retract the corner of the lips. Now, with the rear teeth visible, you can see the six-year molar. It is the sixth tooth from the midline if the child hasn't lost teeth on that side. Study the relationship of the front cusp of the lower molar to the front cusp of the upper molar. Compare the arrangement with that shown in the Angle Classification. Look at the six-year molars. Do they look as if they are meeting correctly (Angle Class I) or like Angle Class II or

Class III? Study the lower cuspid relationship to the upper cuspid. Is it in front or behind? Again, check the Angle Classification illustrations.

6. Look at your child face to face. Ask him to close up and down. Does his mouth open easily and fairly widely, or does he have limited opening? Do you notice any asymmetry as his jaw closes? Does he tend to favor one side and then come back toward the middle as he closes?

If you notice things that don't seem normal or arouse your interest, discuss them with your child's dentist or orthodontist.

As a parent, you are probably interested in knowing when your child should start orthodontic treatment. This varies with each child. The stage of dental development and jaw development help determine the answer. Underdeveloped lower jaws and protruding upper jaws are best treated early when the jaw growth can still be orthodontically guided. Other situations may be started later. Bad habits should be corrected as early as possible.

At the initial examination, your child will have photos, special X rays, and study casts taken. Measurements are checked, and the orthodontist decides on his course of treatment. Now your child is ready for the next step: moving the teeth.

How is tooth movement actually accomplished? Teeth are moved with slow, controlled, or intermittent pressure. The pressure is created with the use of rubber bands, wires, springs, elastic thread, etc. Most tooth movement in the United States is accomplished with some form of bands and/or brackets. The bracket is a shaped piece of metal or plastic, which is either attached directly to the tooth or to a band that is cemented onto the tooth. Then a wire, which is preshaped to the ideal position the teeth should be in, is inserted through the brackets. This is called an *archwire*. It is secured to each of the brackets so it won't slip. Since the teeth are not in the perfect final position yet, the archwire is flexibly distorted as it passes through each bracket. The bracket placement is critical because it will determine, in combination with the archwire, the final tooth position. The wire, now in place but slightly distorted because of the position of the teeth, attempts to straighten back to its original shape (the metal wire has a property which makes its molecules want to return to the original shape when bent). As it tries to

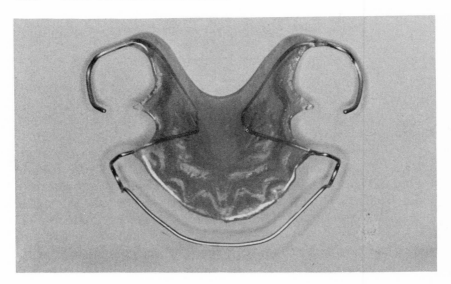

straighten out, it puts pressure on the teeth, and this pressure is transmitted to the bony socket.

That side of the bony socket toward which the tooth is being pushed will melt slightly under pressure, creating room into which the tooth moves. The opposite side of the tooth now has an enlarged space, and new bone is laid alongside the socket wall to close the space to a normal size. This process of bone removal and bone buildup continues while the tooth moves, and for as long as the tooth is receiving active pressure. When it is finally in position, and all other teeth are in position, the archwire becomes passive. At this point, when the orthodontist feels the time has come to remove the brackets and archwire, the patient is given a retainer to wear.

A retainer is usually a plastic-and-wire removable appliance. Its purpose is to keep the teeth fixed in the position into which they have been moved. If the retainer is not worn as prescribed, then the teeth shift and the case begins to relapse. Relapsing means slippage or partial return to the original problem. It can be avoided by following the orthodontist's directions exactly. Failure to follow them is a guarantee that all the time spent will have been in vain.

Before you or your child enter orthodontic treatment, you should know the cost involved and the length of treatment. Once you have decided to enter treatment, definite payment arrangements should be decided on. You should have a plan so that you know and can follow through your obligations, allowing the orthodontist to concentrate on you or your child's dental health. If you have dental insurance, check to see if you have orthodontic coverage. Many orthodontists accept insurance payments, which will make your monthly payments easier. With certain policies, you may have complete coverage.

Tips To Remember

Frequent instructions and considerations for people undergoing orthondontic treatment:

1. Do not eat sweets, sugar, or any of the foods that are decay-producing and could build up around the bands or brackets.

2. After placement of your separators, or bands, you may experience soreness around your teeth. This will go away. If necessary, to help you adapt, take one or two Tylenol or Datril tablets every four hours for pain relief.

3. Follow your orthodontist's directions. If you are wearing a removable appliance, keep it in as often as you are told and for the number of hours necessary.

4. If you have brackets and are using rubber bands, wear the rubber bands as often and for as long as you were told. If you don't, the teeth will not move as fast.

5. Be patient with the strange feelings in your mouth. You will get used to them. It's not for the rest of your life, just a couple of years. Think of how nice you'll look with your new smile.

6. You may not see immediate results because teeth move slowly. Periodically checking with your orthodontist will allow him to review your progress.

7. If your speech is interfered with, practice reading out loud in privacy. You'll improve rapidly.

8. Some tooth looseness is normal during the movement phase.

9. To help prevent decay, keep your teeth clean, especially around the brackets. Use the brush you were given, and use a toothpick carefully between the teeth to prevent gum problems. If you have removable appliances, brush them with your brush and toothpaste.

Again, eliminate soft foods like pretzels, candy, and other sweets, to reduce decay. You might also rinse daily with a fluoride mouthwash to make the enamel surface hard. Last, rinse and irrigate the gums and teeth with a Water Pik or similar irrigator.

10. You may have been told that to get a really good result, it will be necessary to break a habit. Keep trying hard to help the result by doing whatever exercises are necessary, or eliminating any bad habit by avoiding doing it. Remember, you'll be the winner or loser depending on your own ability to follow directions.

11. If something in your mouth breaks, call your orthodontist immediately for an appointment. (Also, see Chapter 15, "Emergencies.")

12. Any removable appliances should always be placed in a container when not being worn. That will prevent them from being lost. If you do lose an appliance, you'll have to pay for a new one because they are made at a laboratory, which charges the orthodontist. He in turn must charge you.

13. After active tooth movement is complete, and you are wearing a retainer, don't give up wearing it prematurely. Retainers may have to be worn up to one year. They should be kept clean, and always returned to their own container when not in the mouth. The suc- ·cess of your case depends on your following the orthodontist's recommendations and not discarding the retainer until he thinks that your new tooth arrangement would not relapse.

14. This is important. Because the gum may get irritated during orthodontic treatment, and may overgrow, causing an overly deep gum space to develop, it is very important at completion of orthodontic treatment that a periodontally-oriented dentist, or even a periodontist, check the gums to see if any minor gum treatment is needed. This may avoid major periodontal breakdown later on.

One Final Note—For Adults

Adult orthodontics is now very popular. If you have a malocclusion, you might discuss with your dentist what could be done with orthodontics. He might be able to treat you, or recommend an orthodontist. Your treatment would generally take less time because unlike an adolescent, your jaws are not growing and your teeth are not still erupting. If you've been self-conscious about your smile or looks, ask your dentist.

Of special interest to some adults is the newer approach to major orthodontic problems with surgery. In recent years surgeons working with orthodontists have refined their procedures so that people with underdeveloped or overdeveloped jaws can be greatly helped. In addition, it's much faster. Where conventional orthodontics might take two to three years, surgical orthodontics may yield the same result or better in ten weeks to five months. Before entering such a course of treatment, I recommend at least two or three separate consultations. Frequently, an oral surgeon and an orthodontist work together as a team. I find that diagnostic differences do exist between different oral surgeon/orthodontist teams. Your dentist will help you make the final choice. You should see your plaster-cast models showing the team's projected final result, so you can envision what their combined efforts will accomplish.

After the oral surgeon completes his work, the teeth are wired together to permit new bone growth and healing. This is similar to the repair of a broken bone in a cast. When those wires come off, final adjustments are frequently made by the orthodontist, and you now have your new mouth, looking much as you had envisioned on the plaster casts shown to you before the operation.

That concludes an overview of the many considerations encountered in the field of orthodontics. Your own perceptiveness, followed by curiosity and interest, should lead you to ask the right questions of your dentist or orthodontist. With your cooperation, or your child's, dramatic dental and facial changes may occur.

DENTAL IMPLANTS, TRANSPLANTS

Although the field of implants is not yet officially designated as a specialty, it is sufficiently distinct and important to present it in this chapter since, unfortunately, some people still lose some or all their teeth.

The area where the teeth were lost is called *edentulous* (without teeth). Your jaw can be partly edentulous, if you're missing a few teeth, or completely edentulous. To replace missing teeth, dentists traditionally have used either fixed bridgework, fixed bridgework with a removable partial, or partial or complete dentures. Today, for the right candidate, there is an alternative called the *dental implant,* which often makes a fixed (nonremovable) bridge possible.

There are basically two types of dental implants: *subperiosteal,* in which the implant rests on bone, and *endosseous,* in which it is *implanted within the bone.* Most implants used today are made either of chrome-cobalt alloy or titanium. Materials being further investigated are ceramics, vitreous and pyrolitic carbon, and plastic polymers.

The Subperiosteal Implant

The most successful kind of subperiosteal implant has been on the lower jaw, where the implant rested on the bone, under the gum. Four or more posts emerge through the gum, and the removable denture fits onto the posts or connector bars. To get the implant to fit correctly, two surgical procedures are necessary. First, the gum is opened to permit an impression of the bone, and later, usually three to six weeks after healing, the gum is reopened and the implant is placed. The technique is more than twenty-five years old and is quite standardized. The success rate is as high as 90 percent.[*] Other types of subperiosteal implants (those used on one side of the jaw and those used on the upper jaw) don't do as well.

These subperiosteal implants are best for patients who just can't tolerate dentures, or whose dentures are painfully pressing on nerve bundles. Before you go ahead with the subperiosteal procedure, your present denture should be carefully examined to make sure it was well made. If not, corrections in fit, or in the bite, should be made. Then you should try to wear the dentures and see if they function better for you. Sometimes a surgical procedure to expose more of your supporting gum ridge will help the denture fit better.

If you have a history of medical problems, especially any uncontrolled severe disease, or diabetes, you may not be a good candidate

[*] W. James Clark, *Clinical Dentistry* (New York: Harper & Row, 1977). Vol. 4, Ch. 46, Ref. 1.

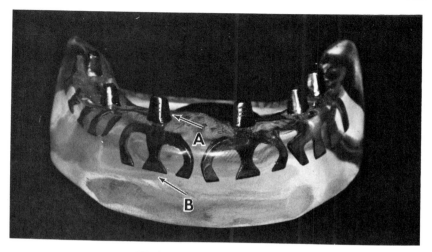

THE SUBPERIOSTEAL IMPLANT

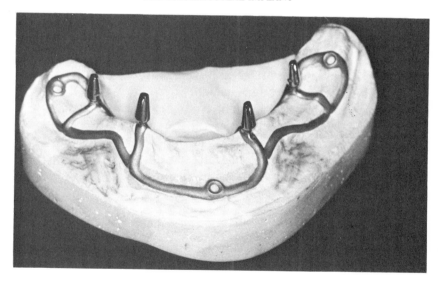

for implants. Your physician should be consulted to evaluate your ability to tolerate the surgery. If you do have an implant, remember that for the implant to be successful, very careful plaque control is necessary, just as with normal teeth.

Last, remember that the implant is a substitute for teeth, to help you chew and function better. It should not be considered inadequate if it doesn't work for you as well as your original teeth did.

The Endosseous Implant (in the bone)

The second type of implant for you to be familiar with is the endosseous type. It looks like the illustrations on page 223. A prime location for this is the lower jaw in the rear, when there are no remaining molar teeth. In the upper jaw, the implant is best placed between remaining teeth. It must be placed into the bone where there is sufficient depth and thickness of bone remaining. In the mouth in the lower jaw it looks like the bottom illustration. The endosseous implant is used most frequently in combination with natural teeth, to replace missing teeth with a fixed bridge rather than a removable partial denture. It has also been used occasionally to replace a lower denture in a person with adequate bone to support a denture, but who really hates taking one in and out of the mouth.

It must be understood that with implants, as with all dental procedures, no guarantees can be given as to how long they'll last. Chances for your success are good if your health is good, and if you intend to be careful and attentive with your oral hygiene.

After placement of the implant, your dentist should see you at very frequent intervals. He will advise you about the frequency of checkups. He wants to make sure that the implant isn't loose, that there is no infection or inflammation, and that the gum is healthy. You should be relatively comfortable to consider your implant successful.

The Endodontic Stabilizer

A third type of implant is the endodontic stabilizer (or endodontic-endosseus implant). It is most typically used to help anchor a tooth—or teeth within a bridge—that is getting loose. It is absolutely critical that there be enough bone without gum pockets left around the root on all sides for this technique to work. Following root-canal therapy, the implant passes through the root of the tooth into the surrounding bone. By extending the length of tooth support

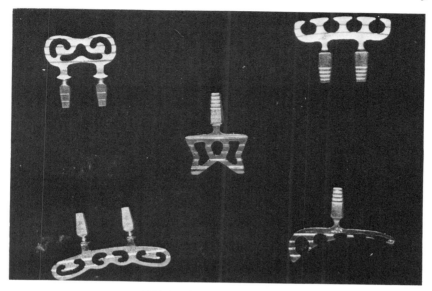

THE ENDOSSEOUS IMPLANT

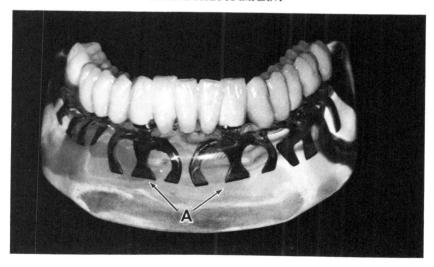

in the bone, it allows you to keep teeth or a bridge that otherwise might require removal. They also can be used as an additional bridge support by placing the implant directly through the bridge in the area of a false tooth.

The Intramucosal Insert

A final type of implant is used to help stabilize upper removable dentures. It is called an *intramucosal insert,* and is used where other types of upper-jaw implants are not feasible. The implants are little button-shaped projections that are attached to the undersurface of the denture. The buttons insert into depressions prepared in the soft tissue of the palate (roof of your mouth). The net result can be a more retentive and stable denture.

ONE DOZEN QUESTIONS ABOUT IMPLANTS AND TRANSPLANTS

1. *What are the main advantages of endosseus implants?*

Endosseus implants provide a useful service for people who have difficulty with removable appliances. Whether the removable is a full denture or a partial denture, it is frequently uncomfortable, or causes gagging, for certain people. If you are one of those, you should investigate the possibility of endosseus implants, which are fixed and would remain in your mouth. It is important that the dentist-implantologist you choose to do the implants be experienced in placing them, and have a good reputation for the end result.

Successful implants provide extra chewing comfort and the psychological satisfaction of knowing that your teeth are not going to be removed and placed in a glass of water.

Implants are used both to save weakened teeth and replace missing teeth. Your appearance and speech may be better than with a denture. In addition, remaining bone support may be preserved longer (just as with real roots) than if your toothless jawbone had to support a denture.

2. *Are implants usually successful?*

Today most implants are successful if the initial diagnosis is carefully made and the patient is felt to be a good candidate, anatomically and psychologically, to receive an implant. Again, the implants should be placed by an experienced practitioner. You might ask him if he is a member of the American Academy of Implant Dentistry, the only national organization at this time which can extensively test and examine its applicants before acceptance for active membership.

3. What are implants made of?

Implants must be biocompatible, i.e., they must be inert in the tissues and not promote rejection mechanisms of the body. The most commonly used materials are titanium, chrome cobalt steel (e.g., vitallium), vitreous carbon, pyrolitic carbon, and ceramics. Plastic polymers are still being studied, but the possibility of their producing cancer remains unresolved.

4. Where are the endosseus implant procedures done?

They are typically done in your dentist's office during regular hours. Any discomfort following the procedure can be adequately handled by prescription medications commonly used to handle pain. Some implant procedures may be completed in one visit; others may require two or three. In addition, there will be a certain number of dental visits to construct the replacement teeth which will fit on the implant. Occasionally, subperiosteal implants are performed in a hospital during a single day's complete operation.

5. Are implants costly?

Cost is always relative. The endosseus implants may cost between $300 and $400, with separate charges for any bridgework and endodontic or periodontal treatment. The subperiosteal implant, which would include both the implant and the superstructure (teeth fitting onto the implant) ranges in cost from $3,500 to $5,000.

6. Who should not have implants?

People with uncontrolled endocrine problems such as diabetes should not have implants. The same is true for any severe metabolic disorder or condition being treated with any medication that could affect the tissue or bone. Generally, any patient who can physically, emotionally, psychologically, and financially undergo extensive bridgework and/or extractions could undergo dental implant procedures. Your individual dentist should help you make the right decision.

7. What may I expect the day the implant is inserted?

You will be anesthetized, the same as for a routine filling. You may experience some soreness or tenderness after the anesthesia wears off. Mild pain relievers will take care of this discomfort. This is more true of the endosseus implant. The subperiosteal may cause more discomfort and swelling, but this too is controlled with proper medication. Such swelling may last for a few days. Usually, the patient leaves the office with temporary teeth attached to, and sitting over the implant. You need not fear walking around toothless. You will be able to smile and speak, even if your chewing requires a little compromise. A soft diet is recommended during this period. After a short period of time (a few days to a few weeks), eating will be more normal.

8. When will the permanent teeth be put in?

Generally they are placed within three to eight weeks. Each patient, as a unique human being, has his or her own particular variations and therefore your own mouth must be considered on an individual basis. Once placed, there will be certain adjustments made by you in chewing, and your dentist may have to adjust your bite before you are comfortable. Eventually, you should enjoy the new stability with which you can eat. Remember that although the implant may function much better than your old denture, it is still not like your normal teeth.

9. How do I care for my teeth now?

Your hygiene must be very good. Bacterial plaque forms around the teeth and the necks of the implants. You should remove it daily with flossing and brushing, and you should also have your teeth cleaned periodically by your dentist.

10. What happens if the implant doesn't work out? How will I know, and what will I do?

If the implant isn't working, it may get loose or it may hurt. Since you should be seeing your dentist regularly, he should see the problem and advise you. If necessary, an implant can be removed and in most cases replaced after a period of time is allowed for healing.

11. How long can I expect the implant to last?

Subperiosteal implants have an excellent track record. They have been in people's mouths as long as twenty-five years and more. Placed on a ridge with the proper type of bone support, and in a patient with a relatively normal medical history, their prognosis is very good.

Endosseous implants have been used with success since the 1960s. They are considered successful when they last five years and beyond. In the beginning they were used everywhere in the mouth, and for many purposes. Today, with greater understanding of where and when they work best, as well as with improvement in design, they are considered to have good longevity, particularly where some natural teeth remain. The presence of natural teeth with adequate bone support, which are attached via bridgework to the implants, reduces the stress on the implant. When the entire case is supported by implants, it receives much greater stress, and is not as likely to hold up as well. Patients with a history of clenching, grinding, or bruxing their own teeth, and who continue to do this with implants, are placing them (as well as any of their own remaining teeth) under greater stress. This may shorten the life of the implant. The same is true if there is any history of uncontrolled diabetes or other health problem that retards healing and repair.

Recently (1978), the National Institute of Dental Research and Harvard University invited fifty experts in oral implantology to a conference to discuss past implant success. As a result of that meeting, the American Dental Association has modified its own view toward implants, and considers the subperiosteal and endosseous implants to be useful adjuncts in rebuilding damaged mouths, when placed using proper guidelines.

Remember, basic periodontal concepts apply even to implants. They must be kept clean, and plaque must be removed daily. Any remaining teeth being used to support endosteal implants should be periodontally healthy or, if they have "pockets," should receive periodontal treatment before the implant is placed. Then the implant is positioned and finally the permanent bridge.

With the above considerations respected, you should find implants of benefit to you, assuming you are a good candidate for them.

12. *What is transplantation?*

Many people think that it is possible to transplant teeth or tooth replicas. In the past, most such attempts have failed because the body rejects them. However, the type of transplantation that has the best chance of succeeding is from the individual's own body. Transplantation of a tooth refers to the transfer, from one site to another, of imbedded, impacted, or erupted teeth which are vital (the nerve is still present) or have been endodontically treated (the nerve has been removed). When this is done within the same individual, it is referred to as *autogenous tooth transplantation.* The tooth may be intentionally removed, treated with root-canal therapy, and then replaced in the socket from which it came. This procedure would be called a *replantation;* actually, *intentional replantation.* This might be necessary if conventional endodontic treatment has failed, and surgical endodontics cannot be performed safely. To be considered successful,* the tooth must remain firm, asymptomatic, and not show any melting away of the root surface or the bone after a minimum of three years.

Transplantation is most frequently used to replace badly decayed first molars with third molars whose roots are incompletely formed.

* W. James Clark, *Clinical Dentistry* (New York: Harper & Row, 1977), Vol. 4, Ch. 9, p. 6.

Because of mixed results over a period of several years, some authorities* prefer extraction of the first molar (if it can't be saved) and placement of a three-unit bridge from second bicuspid to second molar. This way, there is no danger of disturbing formation of the third molar, which might someday be needed in its normal position.

In most cases of tooth transplantation, it is the melting away of the roots which seems to cause the long-term problems. Your dentist must make the choice as to whether such a procedure is advantageous to you.

Unintentional implantation is the procedure used to replace a tooth knocked out accidentally. This may happen when a child falls in sports, or in a fight. If this happens, it is most important to act very quickly. If more than thirty minutes pass before replacement, chances for success diminish. The recommended procedure is for the child, the child's parent, or adult to place the tooth in a sterile gauze bandage or clean handkerchief and keep it cold and moist. Touching the tooth itself should be kept to a minimum and restricted to the crown of the tooth. You must come immediately to the dental office after notifying the dentist so he can get ready for his treatment. You or your child (the injured person) will be anesthetized with local anesthesia and the tooth, after treating the root tip and cleaning the socket, will be placed in the socket as fully as possible. Frequently the patient is asked to guide the tooth back completely. The tooth is then stabilized with a periodontal dressing or immobilized with wire splints.

Arrangements should be made for a tetanus shot or booster, and follow-up appointments arranged. Continued observation will be necessary as long as the tooth is retained.

The last type of implant to discuss is the *heterogeneous transplant*. The heterogeneous transplant consists of artificial teeth—metal, ceramic, carbon, and plastic—placed into the patient's tooth-extraction socket or artificially created sockets. These are still in a clinical trial category, and the field of self-supporting non-at-

* Norman A. Cranin, *The Modern Family Guide to Dental Health* (Briarcliff Manor, N.Y.: Stein and Day, Inc.), p. 312

tached tooth implants is still undergoing extensive testing and evaluation.

As you can see, the field of implants is growing. It holds the promise of improving the chewing ability of people who unfortunately have lost some or all of their teeth earlier in life.

ELEVEN

Oh, My Aching Jaw!
(The TMJ Syndrome)

HAVE YOU EVER heard someone say, "My jaw is killing me!" You might even have had the problem yourself. The pain can be excruciating, like a sharp stab, or just an ache. It usually occurs in the area just in front of the ear opening, and is particularly painful on opening or closing. It can hurt so much that the patient wants to cry. This jaw pain has been referred to as the *temporomandibular joint dysfunction syndrome* or *myofascial pain dysfunction syndrome* (also described in Chapter 10, in section on oral surgery).

The strange aspect of this syndrome is that often aches and pains in other parts of the body are also caused by an inflamed or pathologic jaw joint. For example, headaches, earaches, ringing, buzzing, clicking, popping, and scraping noises in the ears, stiff or aching neck or upper back muscles, shoulder pains, and other upper body/neck/head problems have been traced to primary problems in the jaw joint itself.

Just what is the temporomandibular joint, and what causes the joint to become troublesome? The joint is bilateral—that is, you have one TMJ on each side of your head, just internal and in front of your ear opening. It is a very unusual joint in that it is really composed of two compartments separated by a relatively flat or saucer-shaped cartilage called a *disc*. In each joint, the lower compartment houses the head of the lower jawbone. This jaw bone is U-shaped, and where it rises up on each side to end, under the ear, the ends are shaped like a potato or ball. On each side, this shape rests on the undersurface of the disc in the lower compartment. The upper compartment is formed by the top of the disc and the undersurface

231

of the upper jaw. The entire complex of upper and lower compartments and the disc is encased in a tubular ligament called the *capsule*.

Because your right and left joint are connected to each other via the lower jawbone, they do not function independently of each other. A problem in one joint may easily lead to overcompensation by muscles controlling the jaw movements on the other side of the face.

Normally, when the muscles and joints are functioning in balance, the ball-shaped endings of the lower jaw may slide side-to-side within the joint, or move forward together, or arc downward like a hinge when the jaw opens. Any or all of these motions, and other combinations, are possible in health.

Whenever you chew, talk, yawn, swallow, sing, whistle, or use your mouth, you are involved in some movement of the lower jaw and the joint. To understand how this balanced system becomes unbalanced, there are a few more facts you should know. The upper jaw does not move at all. It is fused to, and is a part of, the skull. We said earlier that the lower jaw does move. What connects these two jaws? In addition to the capsular ligament described earlier, which connects the ball-shaped endings of the lower jaw to the undersurface of the upper jaw, the muscles of mastication (the chewing muscles) all act together to form a muscular sling, which helps hold the lower jaw in proper relation to the upper jaw.

When your jaws are in their normally relaxed position, there is a space between the upper and lower jaws. Dentists call this space the *freeway space*. When dentures or teeth are constructed and placed in the patient's mouth, this space should never be eliminated by opening the bite too much. If the bite is too "open," it may easily lead to TMJ pain. When you wish to close your mouth from a normal rest position, some of your chewing muscles contract. This closes the jaw. If either the muscles, or ligaments which control the delicately balanced system, are overstretched, too slack, inflamed, or in spasm, you may be in great pain. This pain is the TMJ syndrome to which we referred earlier, and may be felt in or near the joint, or in other areas a bit removed that are influenced by nerve signals from the brain responding to problems in the joint.

What causes this problem? In most cases it is a combination of two factors: a bad bite and stress. The bad bite may be caused by a high filling, a twisted or tilted tooth, a shifting of teeth because of not replacing a missing tooth with a bridge, an undererupted or overerupted tooth, or a poor arrangement of several or all teeth when you close them together. What happens in trying to close properly is that the teeth of the lower jaw try to find the most comfortable position of maximum closure. Since cusps of teeth frequently have inclined planes on their biting surfaces, and since the teeth are fixed very solidly in the jaw, a faulty inclined-plane relationship of lower cusps to upper cusps can actually cause the lower jaw to shift to one side or the other as it searches for a comfortable closed position. As the jaw deviates from a symmetrical arrangement, the muscles and ligaments on one side of the joint may be overly stretched, and they tend to compensate by contracting. A struggle is set up between the teeth and their desired closure position, and the ball-socket arrangement of the lower to the upper jaw. This struggle may induce muscle spasm, leading to pain.

WHAT TO DO

If you have this problem, what should you do? First, ask your dentist to help you. He will examine your bite and see if there is a deflecting surface where your teeth are meeting incorrectly. He may adjust the teeth surfaces with high-speed burs or diamond stones. This is called *equilibration* or *bite adjustment*. Very frequently, this may be all that is needed to give relief to the spastic muscles, thus eliminating the referred pain. A very fine knowledge of occlusion (how the teeth meet) is needed to recognize any discrepancies in the bite, as they may be very subtle. Sometimes the bite cannot be corrected by equilibrating because the biting surfaces of the teeth need to be rebuilt. If this is your situation, the dentist may recommend onlays or crowns as he restores your bite to healthy occlusion. At times, orthodontic treatment may be necessary to realign the teeth, and this alone may correct the faulty bite. Or orthodontics followed by occlusal restoration may be indicated. Once the relationship of the inclined planes of the cusps are properly related, jaw to jaw, the muscular spasms frequently disappear.

What if your muscles are already in spasm? What if you find great difficulty in opening your mouth? There are several approaches that your dentist—or the person he refers you to—may use. Heat treatment helps relieve muscle cramping. An electric blanket or hot water bottle applied to the afflicted area, used intermittently, may help. Stretching exercises, done slowly (e.g., opening the jaw and holding it open for a count of ten before closing) may help. Another suggested exercise is to sit at a table with one elbow on the table top and your hand in a fist, rest your lower jaw on the fist and try to open and close your mouth slowly several times. These exercises, done repeatedly several times a day, will restretch cramped, spastic muscles and ligaments. Sometimes the professional treating you will spray the affected area with a very cool spray (ethyl chloride) or inject the area with a dental anesthetic like novocaine (lidocaine is used today), or he may inject saline (salt in water). These act to break the spasm.

In addition, a tranquilizer or muscle relaxant is frequently prescribed to help you relax and, in turn, to ease the tension on the affected muscles. This regimen may continue for a period of several weeks until you are able to open your mouth more completely. Librium, Valium, and Robaxin are the most frequently prescribed. You should only take them for a short time, to avoid becoming dependent on these medications.

Once you are more comfortable, or comfortable enough for your dentist to take study models of your mouth, he may make an appliance of wire and plastic for you to wear. It is called an *auto-repositioner,* or occasionally it is a "Hawley" type of repositioner. Its purpose is to disengage the lower cusps from the upper cusps and allow your jaw to close as a simple hinge. By freeing jaw motion from cusp guidance, the joint has a chance to function in its most natural position and thus begin to heal. These appliances are comfortable, easy to wear, and are made either to fit on the upper or lower jaw, depending on the appliance used.

Your nutrition, especially your need for a balanced diet, is very important during this period. When in stressful situations, one frequently metabolizes much more of the B-complex group of vitamins, as well as vitamin C. Therefore, please review Chapter 4 (covering nutrition) and make sure that you are doing everything you can for yourself as you rebuild your nerves and general health.

What help is available if you are in extreme pain? A qualified professional may choose to inject cortisone or a similar anti-inflammatory agent directly into the joint. This will reduce the inflammation temporarily, but cortisone is not a permanent cure.

In chronic cases, irreversible changes may have occurred to the ligaments, disc, or bony surfaces within the joint. These include arthritis, as well as erosion of bone surfaces and formation of scar tissue. For patients with anatomic changes causing great pain or discomfort, if none of the more conservative approaches work, surgery may be the only answer. You should have multiple consultations and research this approach most carefully before considering TMJ surgery, because you can't undo the surgery there once it is done.

Many dentists have associated stress as one of the most important contributing elements in TMJ syndrome. Therefore, you should carefully reexamine your present situation and determine what stress factors exist, and how they might be eliminated. Is your tension work-related or possibly marital? Have you considered seeing a good psychiatrist or psychologist for counseling? Are you able to discuss your problems with some qualified professional and get aid in that area? Frequently, patients under stress unconsciously try to reduce tension levels by bruxing (grinding or rubbing their teeth at night). Habits like clenching, grinding, or bruxing are particularly harmful to the biting surfaces of teeth because they cause an unnaturally rapid wear. This in turn may bring about cusp or biting surface interference between lower and upper jaw. If this occurs, then the TMJ syndrome may develop secondarily to the bruxing. But if the bruxing continues once the joint pain is present, the pain and muscle spasticity may be very bad. Psychological counseling, relaxants, and dental help may be all needed to correct this situation.

Some newer fields that offer both diagnostic and therapeutic help in treating the TMJ problem include applied kinesiology, to assist in diagnosing the problem, and biofeedback machines, to help you learn how to relax and eliminate negative clenching and grinding habits.

Since the initial cause of the problems may have been a bad bite, it is important that you have your bite checked periodically, even if you are not suffering from this syndrome. Similarly, if you or your child have an open bite, either in front or on the side, you should inquire into both its dental correction and how to stop the tongue-thrusting habit that frequently leads to an open bite. Speech therapists, orthodontists, and personnel called *myofunctional therapists* may help you reeducate your tongue placement, or your child's, during swallowing. Although most adults do swallow properly, bracing the tongue on the roof of the mouth, if you find that you or your child are pressing your tongue against the front teeth when swallowing, you have a problem and you should check into correcting it if at all possible. Malocclusions resulting from tongue thrusts, when coupled with stress, certainly could trigger a TMJ syndrome.

Although most TMJ patients are adults, it is possible for the condition to develop at an early age. Headaches, stuffy ears, earaches or ringing, and clenching or bruxing of the teeth can start as soon as there are teeth in the mouth.

Because of the great variety of symptoms associated with TMJ syndrome, it has been called "the great masquerader." Your dentist is your first line of help. Two other sources for further investigation would be TMJ clinics or a dentist specializing in TMJ problems.

There are TMJ clinics in the following states, and may be others with which I am not familiar.

> *California:* University of California at Los Angeles (UCLA)
>   University of Southern California (USC)
> *Illinois:* University of Illinois
> *New York:* Columbia University
> *Pennsylvania:* University of Pennsylvania

For dentists concentrating in problems of the TMJ, write to:

> The American Academy of Craniomandibular Orthopedics
> 3366 Park Avenue
> Wantagh, NY   11793

The Academy of Stress and Chronic Diseases
c/o Dr. Louis Rigali
610 South Street
Holyoke, MA   01040

TWELVE

The Most Frequently Asked Dental Questions—and Answers

YOU'VE NOW LEARNED a great deal about the mouth, how it breaks down, and how it's repaired. Some of the questions you originally had on your mind have probably been answered; others have not. There are certain questions that occur most frequently regarding one's mouth. Let's consider those questions before going on to the remaining chapters. First we'll discuss questions about teeth, then about gums, and later, about the mouth and joints in general.

TEETH QUESTIONS

Am I getting cavities because my teeth are soft, or because bad teeth run in the family?

If you are getting frequent cavities, you must consider several possibilities. First, your diet may be much too high in sweets. Next, your brushing and flossing techniques may be poor, and perhaps you are not removing the bacterial plaque daily that causes decay.

Another possibility is that all decay from a previous cavity wasn't removed, and a filling was placed that now has decay under it. This may not be your fault. It may or may not be the dentist's, depending on how careful he was originally.

Unless you have been told by your dentist that there is a specific genetic or early formative defect in the formation or mineralization of your teeth, be prepared to accept your responsibility for the condition of your teeth. If they're bad, it's almost always your fault. Try discussing with your dentist what approaches you can take to improve your diet, and to learn preventive techniques. Also, reread chapters 2, 3, and 4, if you are still unsure.

Do I have to lose my teeth because my parents did?

In most cases, the answer is no. Most bad teeth are not inherited, but are caused by neglect, improper diet, poor cleansing habits, and not visiting your dentist for early examination and repair.

How do you find a good dentist?

A good dentist should not just be a "nice man" or a "nice woman." In Chapter 6 we discuss choosing a new dentist. Basically, if you understand the material in this book, you will know what a good dental examination consists of. This will help you know if you're being given one. You can also judge by whether your dentist seems progressive, and is involved in helping you control, reduce, or eliminate your dental disease. If he doesn't teach prevention, and doesn't give you any dietary instruction, and always tells you "things are fine, what a great mouth you have," you might consider a second opinion. For your sake, I hope he's right and your mouth *is* terrific, but it's always good to be certain you're getting a very careful, detailed examination. This helps prevent major problems later in life.

My dentist recommended gold onlays for certain teeth. What's an onlay, and why can't I get a silver filling?

An onlay is a good restoration used to not only replace missing tooth structure, but to help strengthen the cusps of the teeth. It does this not only by holding the inner surfaces of the biting table of rear teeth but also by extending slightly onto the tongue and cheek sides of the tooth. This helps prevent the weakened tooth from splitting if excess force results from chewing.

Silver fillings don't provide this extra strength. They fill, but they don't support. So, if your tooth has had previous fillings and is no longer too strong, or if the decay is fairly extensive, an onlay may be the best restoration, even though it costs more.

When do I need a crown?

The most frequent reason for having a crown made is because the tooth is so broken down that any other restoration might lead to a fracture of the tooth. A crown supports the tooth because it completely encircles it, holding it tightly all around the neck of the tooth. Another reason for getting a crown (on a front tooth) would be to improve your appearance. Last, if you have one or more missing teeth, each remaining tooth that your dentist uses for support for a new fixed bridge will receive a crown. Here each crown will be joined to its neighbor to comprise the bridge.

How long should a crown last?

A well-made crown, fitting tightly, on a tooth with good periodontal support and no periodontal pockets, could easily last fifteen to twenty years. To help maintain your crowns as long as possible, you should follow the plaque-control instructions already given, to reduce the possibilities of tooth decay at the crown margin, and gum disease where the crown slips under the gum.

Why is the gum around my porcelain jacket a darker color than the other gum?

There are two possible reasons. First, when the porcelain-jacket crown was made, the tooth was prepared, or drilled, too close to the connection between gum and tooth. When the crown was placed, it squeezed, and is still squeezing the tissue. This leads to poor circulation, or cyanosis of the tissue. The bluish or darker color indicates the pooling of stagnant blood and waste products.

Another possible reason is recession. If your gum has receded slightly, you may be noticing the difference between the edge of the porcelain jacket and the root that is visible before it disappears into the gum, or you may be seeing the metal edge of a veneer crown or ceramic crown. Both the darker root, and certainly the edge of metal from the veneer or ceramic crown, could show as a dark line.

How does "capping" teeth affect the gums?

If the "caps" are well done and fit passively into the gum space without pressing into the gum lining, there should be no irritation. In addition, that portion of the cap that inserts into the gum space must be very thin. If the cap is too bulky, the gum will be affected. If the cap is improperly made, the gum may become inflamed, hurt, feel sore, or bleed easily. Ask your dentist to make another crown if you find these problems after insertion of a new crown. Normally, a properly made crown will not harm the tissue, and should protect and strengthen the tooth.

Do impacted wisdom teeth always have to be removed? What about wisdom teeth fully erupted in the mouth?

Impacted wisdom teeth do not always have to be removed. If they are embedded totally in the bone and do not have any abnormalities surrounding them (such as a cyst), they may be left in and checked with X rays every eighteen months. If they are partially erupted, then they may present a problem. Frequently, the eruptive force of the wisdom tooth presses on teeth in front of it and causes changes in their alignment. Sometimes a tissue flap lying over the partially erupted wisdom tooth gets infected because of trapped food and bacteria. Occasionally, a deep periodontal pocket may develop between a wisdom tooth and the second molar in front of it. In the above situations, it would generally be best to extract the wisdom tooth. Once one wisdom tooth on one side of the face is extracted, the opposing tooth is best removed to prevent supereruption, which could cause periodontal problems and bite problems.

What causes stains on teeth?

Stains may be caused by certain bacteria, and may be brown, green, black, or even orange. Smoking causes stains, and so do coffee, tea, and certain other beverages. All these stains can be reduced or sometimes eliminated by proper brushing and flossing. Do not use an extremely abrasive toothpaste for a prolonged period of time to remove stains. You may thin out the enamel of the tooth. It would be better to eliminate the cause of the staining. If the stains still persist after your best efforts, you may need a thorough cleaning from your dentist or hygienist.

What's the best way to keep my teeth white?

Brushing and flossing correctly, and using a good toothpaste that is approved by the American Dental Association. Again, avoid toothpastes that are too abrasive, because they may wear away some of the enamel.

Can my teeth shift again after braces are removed?

Yes, although the amount of shift usually is not too much. To prevent this shift, normally you are advised to wear a retainer, which is a thin plastic appliance with a bracing wire attached, to keep your teeth in their final position. You should wear the retainer until your dentist or orthodontist advises you to discontinue.

I'm afraid of damage from X rays. Will they hurt me, produce cancer, or damage my reproductive organs?

No. Assuming your dentist is using modern X-ray machines, the amount of radiation from X rays reaching the more sensitive parts of the body (e.g., reproductive organs) is about the same as that received daily from natural sources, such as atmospheric X rays. If you're concerned, it's a good idea to ask your dentist how many total seconds of X-ray exposure you're getting. For a full-mouth series of fourteen to twenty films, the total exposure should not be more than between seven and ten seconds to the face. Your neck and the trunk of your body should be covered with a lead apron. Once every three years is frequent enough for a full-mouth series of X rays, if your mouth has not had extensive dental work. If you have had extensive dental work, once every two years would be best to stay on top of the situation.

Why are X rays necessary? Can't he just look in my mouth?

No. There are many diseases and conditions which occur in the mouth and jaws. Some may be life-threatening, and can only be seen on an X ray. In addition, the X ray reveals many important dental findings that influence treatment choices. X rays show impacted teeth, bone loss from periodontal disease, ill-fitting dental restorations, broken roots, abscesses, decay, and inadequate room for tooth eruption, to name just some of the important items seen.

When do I bring my children to a dentist?

Today, the feeling among authorities in children's dentistry is that between two and two-and-one-half years would be best for the first examination. (See Chapter 10, section on pedodontics).

What's a root canal? Does it hurt?

A root-canal treatment is done for a tooth with an infected nerve, and perhaps an abscess at the root tip. Treatment consists of removing the diseased pulp (tissue) from within the tooth, sterilizing the canal in which the tissue normally lives, and filling the resulting empty canal with a material that is compatible with the tissues surrounding the root tip. Usually a series of three or four appointments is needed, and the procedure is done under anesthesia, so you won't feel it. It is best done under a sheet of rubber called a *rubber dam,* to prevent you from swallowing the small instruments used to perform the root-canal treatment. It is an excellent technique for saving a tooth, and as long as there is enough supporting bone around the tooth to warrant keeping it, root-canal treatment is far better for you than pulling the tooth out.

I'm afraid of going to the dentist. Can they knock me out and do it all at once?

Some dentists have taken special training to allow them to treat patients who want to be totally unconscious. There are advantages and disadvantages. The advantages for very fearful patients are that they may have been putting off work for a long time because they were afraid of being hurt. It's much better for such patients to be "put out" rather than having no work done because of their fears.

Since most dentists today are trained in giving topical anesthesia to numb the surface skin of the mouth, followed by a local anesthetic to numb the tooth, if your dentist is gentle, there should be very little pain, and if you can trust your dentist, you won't need to be "put out." If you are very afraid, ask your dentist if he has nitrous oxide (laughing gas), a very harmless and pleasant gas which makes you more detached and helps calm your fears.

What about tooth implants? What are they? Do they work?

When we discuss implants, we are really discussing two types. A natural tooth implant works best if it's a tooth that was knocked out, was immediately saved, washed clean with water but not scrubbed, and brought to your dentist immediately. He may elect to do one of two things. He may either reimplant the tooth and wire or cement it in position; or do root-canal treatment and then wire or cement it in position. After several months, the wires or cement may be removed and the tooth tested for looseness. Decisions are made then regarding the future of the tooth and any further dental treatment or fixation necessary. The faster you get to the office (best would be within thirty minutes of the tooth being knocked out), the less need for a root canal.

There is another type of implant more commonly referred to by adult patients who are missing teeth. This is the metal implant, or carbon implant, which is inserted through an opening in the gum and bone. A portion of the implant is left emerging into the mouth from the gum. Upon this stub, a tooth crown can be built. Usually, several such stubs are used, so that a bridge may be built. Sometimes some stubs are used along with natural teeth. You will find more information in Chapter 10.

GUM QUESTIONS

What's pyorrhea?

Pyorrhea is another name for periodontal disease. "Pyo" means "pus," and "rhea" means "flow." It refers to a flow of pus out of the gum space. For this to happen, the degree of gum infection is usually quite severe and is accompanied by severe bone loss. It tends therefore to be the latest stage of the disease, when teeth may actually have to be extracted. Try not to let your mouth get to that stage, by following the information and instructions in chapters 1, 2, and 3.

Why do my gums bleed?

Gums bleed when the gum lining has broken down, and is ulcerated. You may notice this when brushing, or eating fruit, or using a toothpick or dental floss. If you follow proper plaque-control methods, you can stop the bleeding within a few days. If the bleeding is not stopped, periodontal disease gets worse and may finally cause tooth loss.

If your gums happen to bleed spontaneously, without your even touching them, visit a dentist or physician immediately. A complete blood count should be taken to see if there is anything wrong with your blood. Certain conditions, such as leukemia, frequently show up first in the gum.

What's the best kind of toothbrush?

For most people a three- to four-row soft nylon brush with rounded bristles is best. It permits you to brush in the gum space correctly, as described in Chapter 2.

Is a Water Pik important?

A Water Pik can be helpful, and may help flush out food debris, loose bacteria and cells from between the teeth and in the gum space. It is not a substitute for proper flossing and brushing, and is down from the top of the list as an effective hygiene aid, because it does not remove plaque. Therefore, it can be considered only an auxiliary aid.

What does bad breath come from?

Most bad breath comes from diseased gums or decayed teeth. In addition, smoking increases mouth odor, as does failing to remove plaque daily. Certain foods may contribute if they are not removed from between the teeth. If one has digestive disorders, or eats strong foods such as garlic or onions, this too could contribute. Overwhelmingly, a dirty mouth with diseased gums and rotten teeth is the biggest cause.

How often should I have my teeth cleaned?

This varies from patient to patient. Some people have greater susceptibility to gum breakdown. Others smoke, or drink more coffee or tea. Some people, especially diabetics, may form calculus more quickly. Generally, about once every three months could be used as an average figure. If you're very good with your mouth hygiene, you might only require it once every six months, or once a year. You and your dentist should decide together, based on your dental history and personal plaque-control efforts.

How does my diet affect my teeth? Are any foods especially bad?

Diet can affect your teeth greatly. Foods that contain sugar are particularly harmful, and the more concentrated the sugar the greater the danger. For example, caramels are worse than soda, and soda is much worse than orange juice. Since sugar has also been indicted as a very probable contributor to heart disease, I think that a careful person would do well to avoid sugar. Other foods that are not considered good for teeth are refined carbohydrates. These also may lead to cavities, because the carbohydrate is attacked by bacteria of the mouth and converted to acids, which cause the teeth to decay.

What causes gum recession?

Gum recession generally is caused by excessive brushing, which literally "skins" the gum off the neck of the teeth. It can also be caused genetically, when the actual gum band around the neck of the tooth is too narrow in height. This in turn allows the muscle fibers of the mucous membrane to pull at the gum border during lip and cheek movement, leading over a period of time to gum recession. It occasionally results from a periodontal surgical procedure called a *gingivectomy*, which today among periodontists, is relatively obsolete because it removes too much gingiva (gum). Today we prefer to do "flaps" to preserve the gum.

How can gum recession be repaired?

There are several procedures used today, mainly by surgically trained periodontists, to cover over roots that have had recession. Each problem may require a special solution, and sometimes the gum can't be totally returned to where it was at age fifteen. Nevertheless, it can frequently be improved.

What happens if gum recession isn't treated?

This depends on several factors. For an older person, it might not be significant. For a younger person, or one in midlife, failure to correct an inadequate zone of gum where recession has already occurred can lead to further recession, gum irritation, and root sensitivity, and possibly also contribute indirectly to root decay or bone loss, and perhaps tooth loss.

How often should I go to the dentist?

At least once every six months for a few X rays, cavity check, probing, and cleaning. You would do better, on average, going four times a year, unless your dentist advises you that that frequency isn't necessary. Periodontally, I feel that scalings and curettage on people over thirty should be done at least every three months, unless the patient is very good with plaque control. And it would help if you were checked for periodontal disease with the phase microscope.

What is a night guard?

A night guard is a thin piece of plastic specially formed to fit over your upper or lower teeth. It is worn at night while you sleep. Its purpose is to prevent you from grinding or clenching your own teeth, which could damage the teeth, roots, and supporting bone. When you wear the night guard, if you do grind (or "brux") your teeth at night, you only damage the surface of the night guard.

What causes me to grind my teeth at night?

Grinding may be the result of many factors. Most commonly, it is a manifestation of inner tension or aggression. Infants have been observed, even before teeth enter the mouth, to move their jaws in the same manner that adults do. The infant seems to be satisfying very basic needs of tension reduction by rubbing his lips and gum pads against each other. After teeth erupt, the habit of rubbing to reduce tension may continue, except now the teeth are rubbed against each other, rather than the gum pads.

Another reason for grinding described in the literature is a lack of harmony between tooth intercuspation and joint closure. Here the patient attempts to close comfortably and, not being able to, tries to position his jaw so that his teeth do not slip against each other. If his teeth are slightly out of exactly correct occlusion, his struggle to place them in a comfortable position causes him to keep searching for maximum closure with lower jaw movements. This forward-and-back, or side-to-side, movement, rubbing the teeth against each other is called *bruxing*.

Can bruxing cause damage?

Yes. Teeth can be worn excessively. Sometimes, the temporomandibular joint may hurt, or the pain may be referred to the temples, side of the face, neck, or shoulders.

How is it usually treated?

Most commonly, the patient has a bite adjustment (spot-grinding on the surfaces of the teeth with a bur or stone) or a series of such adjustments, to eliminate obvious slips or interferences. If opening of the jaws is limited, it is sometimes necessary to use a night guard or Hawley bite-plane appliance to break the muscle spasms preventing the jaw from fully opening. After wearing this for several weeks, and sometimes taking a muscle relaxant or tranquilizer in addition, the jaws become sufficiently relaxed to allow for wider opening. At that point, the bite is again checked to eliminate any cusp interference or slips. These are eliminated by selectively grinding the proper marks on the teeth. It should be noted that generally the approach described is treating symptoms, not causes. Underlying tension or aggression may also have to be dealt with, possibly via psychotherapy.

Why is a tooth sometimes sore after a new filling or crown is placed?

Usually because the filling or crown is "high." This means that there is excess metal preventing the opposite tooth from closing down completely on the newly restored tooth when the jaw closes. Treatment would be to adjust the bite on the newly restored tooth and the opposing one until all bite marks on the cusps are in proper position, and the patient is comfortable.

What causes a "toothache"?

A toothache can be caused by decay; by a periodontal pocket; by a fracture or vertical split; by an incorrect biting relationship between that tooth and the opposing one; and by trapped gas under an old filling or crown. Sensitivity is most frequently caused when either the enamel or the covering of the root (the cementum) has been worn through, and the dentine is exposed. Dentine is much more sensitive to heat and cold than the enamel or cementum, and stimulation from heat or cold is experienced as pain or ache.

My teeth are sensitive. Can anything be done about this?

There are several approaches used today. One approach, when possible, is to add a dental material called *composite* to the sensitive area and cover it over. A second approach is for your dentist to use one of several available materials (either fluoride or calcium hydroxide derivatives) on the sensitive areas, and repeat this procedure several times. This stimulates the nerve to lay down more tooth structure to insulate itself from temperature changes. Your dentist might also try the new procedure called ionto phoresis. This has greatly helped people who have experienced it.

Last, should all else fail, a filling may be placed, if the sensitivity is very annoying.

What are the chances of having periodontal disease?

Excellent. Almost guaranteed, if you live long enough, but there is hope if you read and apply Chapters 1, 2, 3, and 5.

What causes canker sores?

Canker sores are small, white ulcers that occur on the mucous membrane tissues of the mouth. They are usually found on the inner lip, the lining of the cheek, and the undersurface of the tongue. They are painful and usually last from one to two weeks. They have been associated with allergy to citrus fruits, and are also thought to be the possible result of a delayed hypersensitivity to a mouth bacterium. At this time, the exact cause is still unknown. The best treatment I have found for this problem is to rinse the mouth with a good mouthwash, then dry the sore with a Q-Tip, and then place denture adhesive paste over the sore. This seems to accelerate the healing greatly. In addition, get lots of rest and eat properly. The sores should go away within a few days. Canker sores are also known as *aphthous ulcers.*

What are cold sores?

Cold sores, also called "herpes," are caused by a virus known as the herpes simplex virus. There are actually a family of herpes viruses. Those affecting man fall into two distinct groups, Type 1 and Type 2. Type 1 strains usually cause infections of the mouth, lips, and oropharynx. Type 2 strains are responsible for infections of the genitals.

Herpes simplex Type 1 occurs in two forms: primary and recurrent. The primary attack with clinical symptoms usually occurs in infants after the age of six months. It may occur in adolescents and adults. The most common clinical symptom is an acute inflammation of the gum and mouth tissues. It occurs in less than 1 percent of children. The most frequent age of occurrence is from one to three years, with fourteen months being the most common. Prior to onset, there may be irritability, fever, and a sore throat. Then the gum and mucous membranes may become very red and swollen. There may be lesions that burst and become ulcers. This acute stage lasts about seven days.

After one or more exposures to the virus, a balance is established between the human host and the latently active but permanently established virus. When host resistance is reduced, the virus breaks out. It is recognized as "cold sores" or fever blisters. The outbreak has been associated with trauma, allergy, menstruation, sunburn, emotional upset, and fever. Carriers can spread the virus. The most common site for recurrence is the junction of the inner lip with the outer lip. The early indications of an outbreak are a slight swelling and a burning sensation, followed by a little blister. Besides the lips, another common site is the hard palate. Thre is no known treatment other than rest, good nutrition, and elimination of stress, to give the body a chance to recover and repair.

THIRTEEN

Secrets of an Attractive Smile

NATURALLY, YOUR APPEARANCE is very important to you. Your smile and your profile play a big part in whether you are pretty, handsome, or pleasing to other people. Your good looks, in turn, are dependent on many factors: skeletal relationships, skeletal proportions, dental relationships, muscle balance, facial relationships, genetics, and so on.

We tend to take our looks for granted. We may not like them, but usually we learn to live with them. We frequently don't realize how easily they can be improved. It does take a trained eye to identify the problem and recommend the proper solution. Your dentist can be of great help to you in recognizing malrelationships and in arriving at suggestions for improvement. The first problem to analyze is whether the malrelationship is dental or skeletal, or perhaps facial or muscular. Let's suppose that it is skeletal. What can be done?

SKELETAL PROBLEMS IN JAW RELATIONSHIPS

Some people have profiles like gophers and others have lantern jaws. The section on oral surgery in Chapter 10 explains how these malrelationships can be corrected. What is important for you to know is that if you do have a protruding upper or lower jaw, or an undersized one, and if you always wished that you could look more normal, this may indeed be possible. You will need a consultation with an orthodontist and an oral surgeon to determine whether your problem requires just orthodontic therapy, or whether you may also need an oral surgeon's assistance. Together, they will determine, by analyzing your jaw-to-skull relationship, where changes should be made, and with what techniques.

As with any building, when you're improving the structure you have to start with the foundation. Although most people think of just rearranging teeth, it is really the skeletal relationships that first should be studied. It may turn out that the problem is only dental, which makes it easier to solve. In Chapter 10, the sections on orthodontics and oral surgery explain how your problem can be corrected if it is truly skeletal, and how cephalometric studies (special X rays) help provide the answer.

DENTAL PROBLEMS

If the problem with your teeth and smile is only dental, there are several different approaches that can be used, depending on the dental problem. Let's look at some common problems and see how they are solved.

Discolored Teeth

Teeth may be discolored because of stains on their surface, or because of internal changes within the tooth. Common causes of external, or surface, discoloration are bacterial deposits, tartar, cavities, and old fillings. Solutions here are obvious. Your teeth should be cleaned and polished. Any old fillings that are stained, discolored, or leaking should be replaced.

There are some discolorations that occur within the tooth. White, chalky patches may be due to hypocalcification, or to having been exposed to excess fluoride, usually from the water supply, during the time the teeth were calcifying. Two possible solutions, if your teeth are extremely unattractive to you because of discoloration, are bonding or capping.

BONDING   Bonding is a technique in which a polished tooth is etched with buffered phosphoric acid, and then a plastic-like, tooth-colored material called *composite resin* is added to the etched area. Bonding is particularly helpful for younger patients, because it improves appearances without requiring all the tooth structure to be reduced, as with porcelain jackets. Although greatly improving esthetics, bonding does not offer the esthetic perfection of full porcelain jackets. It is frequently necessary to use bonding for a younger person's tooth when the pulp of the tooth is still large and the dentist wishes to avoid grinding the tooth down, thereby injuring the pulp. Similarly, the conservative bonding technique, by not injuring the pulp, will allow the root to form completely. This conservative approach helps avoid root-canal treatment. A few years later, it may be possible to bond again, or to make a porcelain jacket because the tooth is fully formed. Your dentist can guide you with the appropriate solution.

Another type of discoloration, usually resulting from trauma to the tooth due to an accident, is a dark tooth. This darkness is due to bleeding within the tooth at the time of the accident. As time goes by, the dried blood decomposes, resulting in a brownish or grayish black color.

The solution to this problem is to have a root canal done and then bleach the tooth, which will whiten it, or to have root-canal treatment, followed by a post-crown (a post internally builds up the tooth, and a crown is placed over it to look like a natural tooth).

Some other common problems that you might find in your mouth are chipped teeth, teeth worn out at the biting edges, pitted teeth, or teeth with notches near the gum line. These problems may sometimes be treated by simple slight reshaping of the tooth by your dentist. To do this, he uses special high-speed burs and stones. In addition, he may also use bonding.

CAPPING   If you are an adult, and your teeth are properly aligned, but perhaps are badly chipped, or have been filled too many times and show stains and changes in color between tooth and filling material, then "jackets" or crowns may be for you. For front teeth, the two most frequently used restorations are either porcelain-fused-to-metal crowns or porcelain jackets. Of the two, porcelain-fused-to-metal crowns are stronger, but not quite as naturally esthetic. They are nevertheless very good. For the most natural esthetics, where possible to use them, dentists recommend porcelain jackets. Because they have no metal supporting the porcelain, they are more translucent and natural. Where individual teeth are to be capped, are periodontally strong, and the bite is not traumatic, porcelain jackets are the restoration of choice for front teeth.

You might also consider crowning some of your teeth if you have:

1. Badly decayed teeth
2. Teeth that are very worn down
3. Teeth with badly fractured edges
4. Teeth that have had root-canal treatment (to help strengthen the tooth)
5. Misshapen or malformed teeth

You should be aware that crowning a tooth is not a step to be taken lightly. If you can restore the tooth with bonding, that will be much more gentle to both the tooth and surrounding gum tissue. Crowns don't usually last a lifetime—unless you're already on in years. They may average ten years, though they could last much longer, but may have to be replaced someday, either because of decay under the crown or shrinkage of the gum, creating an esthetic problem.

Of the various crown types being used today, other than porcelain jackets, porcelain-fused-to-gold—or to other nonprecious metal alloys—is the most aesthetic. An earlier type of crown, the acrylic veneer, is also still used in certain situations. Esthetics here are good at the beginning, but acrylic does stain and wear out much more rapidly than porcelain.

Sometimes patients complain that a crown or cap looks like a false tooth, not like "nature's own." It is difficult to reproduce natural teeth perfectly, but this is where the artistic ability of your dentist comes in. His skill at carving the porcelain tooth when it comes to him from the laboratory will play a great role in achieving a natural look. You should know that the shape of the crowned tooth plays a greater role in a lifelike appearance to the tooth than does color.

If the shape is good, then the color is the other key factor that can make or break the esthetic effect. The light used by your dentist to select the right color and shade is most important. One of the best lights available today is a color-corrected fluorescent bulb made by Verd-A-Ray Corporation. It is actually called "Indoor Sun."

Summing up the individual crown, if your tooth is broken down, the crown is the restoration of choice, and can be made to look life-like if your dentist follows the proper procedures in both shaping the tooth and choosing the color and shade.

Esthetics and Missing Teeth—Or Poorly Done Bridgework

What can you do about missing teeth, or old bridgework, or small removable bridges (partials)?

When you smile, if you show a missing tooth, you certainly should consider getting a bridge. If your old bridge is showing excessive wear, or your gums have receded, showing the darkened root structure underneath, you may also need a new bridge. Also if the shape or length of the teeth on your old bridge was not exactly to your liking, you might consider replacing that bridge with a more modern one. The replacement of the missing tooth or teeth should be with a new porcelain-fused-to-metal bridge. Recent improvements in laboratory technology, as well as greater knowledge regarding periodontal health and crown contour, now permit the dentist to obtain excellent esthetic results. Considerations are similar to those of a single crown.

Today, your dentist knows how to place the margin of the crown more exactly into the gum space without digging too deeply into the gum attachment. When crowns and bridges are very carefully made, there is little or no gum irritation, and your gum looks pink and healthy. *If you have puffy gums around your old bridge, it may be time for your dentist and periodontist to help restore the tissue and teeth to a better state of health.*

An important point for you to understand is that if there is any gum inflammation, or any periodontal disease, it *must* be treated and eliminated *before* any capping is done. It is very sad for a patient to pay good money for "caps" without periodontal treatment, and still have puffy gums or pockets. If the patient then seeks periodontal treatment, frequently the gum line is moved away from the cap, exposing the metal edge. Obviously, if the smile shows the metal edge, and this had happened to you, you'd be upset. The moral of the story is: Get the gums healthy before you cap the teeth!

SPECIAL ESTHETIC PROBLEMS OF
TEETH—SPACING, PROTRUSION, ETC.

What can be done about the following problems?

1. You have a space between your front teeth.
2. Your front teeth stick out.
3. Your front teeth are crowded.
4. Your front teeth tip back in and you show too much gum.
5. Your upper front teeth extend deeply over your lower front teeth. You find that your lower front teeth can barely be seen when you smile, and you bite into the palatal tissue behind your upper teeth.

All of the above, and many other combinations and situations, are problems that an orthodontist—or a dentist well trained in orthodontics—can help solve. The result for you will be a much prettier or handsome smile. If a general dentist undertakes treatment, it is important for him to know whether your case is indeed a simple one, or requires complex tooth movements. Therefore, his analysis for you should include the use of study models, X rays, and perhaps a special X ray called a cephalogram, to help establish the diagnosis. As treatment continues and changes occur, he can use the earlier data to analyze your progress.

Did you know that it is possible to correct a malocclusion (bad bite) anytime during one's life, as long as there is enough bone around the teeth? Orthodontics is not just for children. Frequently, one sees adults with spacing between their front upper teeth. This may be a purely orthodontic problem, with the amount of bone supporting the teeth fairly normal. More frequently a person with this problem is suffering from periodontal breakdown, tipping of rear teeth, and drifting and protrusion of the front teeth—causing spacing. This type of patient can be helped with a combination of orthodontics, periodontal treatment, and reconstruction of the bite with capping. If periodontal treatment alone is done for such a case, and the teeth are not tipped into a better position, then pressures from the bite may loosen these teeth further. Capping (reconstruction) will help stabilize the teeth, but ideally, before any capping, teeth should be brought into a better relationship over the jawbone with orthodontics. Successful clinical results reported by many dentists over the years have demonstrated the soundness of the combined perio-ortho-prosthetic approach for the periodontal patient with collapsed bite and protruding front teeth.

Orthodontists and general dentists doing orthodontics frequently use removable appliances, elastic thread, or direct bonding of plastic, tooth-colored brackets to the teeth to achieve their results. In recent years, because of these new techniques, many adults have improved their smile, their bite, and the longevity of their teeth. So if you don't like the way your teeth look, discuss possible corrective measures with your dentist.

HEALTHY, ATTRACTIVE GUMS FOR AN ATTRACTIVE SMILE

You may not have thought about it much, but if your gum line is not well related to your lips and teeth, it can be the cause of an ugly or unpleasant smile. There are many conditions of the gum tissue that could cause this. Your gum might be red, swollen, and inflamed. It may have receded. It may be bulbous and lie too much over your teeth hiding part of them from view. The causes of these problems may be your mouth hygiene; they might be improperly designed dental work that crowds the gum tissue, making it impossible for you to clean in between your teeth; or your crowns may intrude too deeply into the gum space, irritating the tissue. Improperly designed crowns are major gum irritants. So, too, are plaque and calculus. The solutions to these problems are first to identify the cause and then correct it.

If your gum is red, swollen, and spongy because you're not into plaque control and gum massage (compression with a Perio-Aid or Stim-U-Dent), you'll have to learn these techniques (Chapter 2). If you're doing your hygiene homework well, and you're still having problems next to a crown or crowns, get an opinion from your dentist, and perhaps a second opinion from another dentist or periodontist, as to whether your crowns are the irritants. They may require replacement.

If, after learning to do plaque control and tissue compression, your gums still look puffy, or too large, or extend over your teeth, your dentist or periodontist should treat the gums with the proper periodontal procedure. You might require curettage, a gingivectomy, flap surgery, or electrosurgery. Any of these techniques might be needed to bring the tissue back to a healthy normal shape and contour. Gum tissue should be pink, firm, and flat.

There are two other special problems of interest regarding your gum line: (1) recession showing the roots; (2) high lipline showing too much gum.

Recession can be treated in many situations with a grafting procedure in which gum tissues (or tissue with the same characteristics as gum) is placed over the exposed tooth root. Part of the tissue covers the exposed root, and the rest is adapted to the adjacent tissue so that it has a blood supply and a tissue base with which to join. These grafts, called *free soft-tissue autografts* (or *free gingival grafts*), work very well. They stop further recession and frequently can be used to partly cover bare roots. When the problem is only on a single tooth, gum tissue adjacent to that tooth frequently can be slid over to hide the defect. This is a laterally repositioned graft.

The last problem to discuss is that of the high lipline and low gum line. You may see someone look like the illustration on page 260. The problem here is a very gummy smile. This can be corrected by surgically raising the gum line (frequently the periodontist also raises the underlying bone by one eighth inch and then brings the gum up to it, suturing it in position). Next, the edges of the teeth are shortened. Sometimes the teeth are capped. The net result is to bring the gum line and body of the upper teeth closer to the upper lip to provide a more natural smile. This greatly increases the attractiveness of the smile.

So far, we've talked about the shape of your jaws, the position of your teeth, problems with teeth, old dental work, and last, having healthy gums. There is one other mouth area to be aware of when thinking of your smile . . . your lips. The shape of your lips is partly

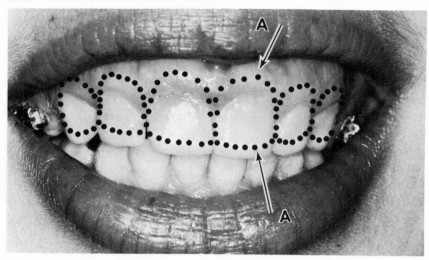

AN EXAMPLE OF A HIGH LIPLINE AND LOW GUMLINE

determined genetically. Yet how they lie against your teeth when in a state of rest, or when smiling, is very much related to the shape and degree of fullness of the entire front group of teeth. If your teeth protrude too far, your lips may not close. If your teeth tip back inwards, your face may have a flat appearance. If your upper teeth extend out too far over your lowers, your lower lip may catch between the upper and lower teeth. Or you may have a habit of placing your lower lip under your upper teeth when you're tense or contemplating something. This can cause a further protrusion of your upper teeth and give you that "Bugs Bunny" look. The dentist to see for these problems is again our friendly orthodontist. He will help you correct any harmful habits while rearranging the relationship of the teeth, so that your teeth allow your lips to drape over them in a pleasing manner.

Some people have excess lip tissue, or a cleft lip that was repaired in childhood. Frequently, these two esthetic problems can be improved through the skills of a plastic surgeon so as to eliminate unnecessary lip tissue, or remodel and reshape tissue that is not relating correctly. If you do have a problem with your lip tissue, I suggest that you consult at least two plastic surgeons to find out what solutions do exist.

Frankly, I would like to restate a thought that I originally got from Dr. Maxwell Maltz in his book *Psycho-Cybernetics*. Looking good may help one to feel good, but positive self-image is all-important. Our internal level of confidence, our inner security, the strength of our egos, has much to do with our satisfaction regarding our looks. We can be average-looking but feel good about ourselves, and from this inner self-confidence we may look good to the world. Or we can be beautiful and handsome externally and project such a miserable personality that others think of us as being "ugly." Looks are important; they may give us extra confidence. But the inner beauty of a relaxed, assured, positive personality is equally important in how you look to others.

FOURTEEN

New Techniques for Pain Control

THERE ARE MANY things to understand in examining the question of pain and pain control. For example, the degree of pain you feel is not really measurable in absolute terms, but is highly subjective. How you feel about dental pain or dental sensation varies with your anxiety or fear level. It varies because of your prior dental experience. If you had a warm, gentle, careful dentist in your early years, you may be relatively relaxed today as you await your dentist's recommended procedure. If you had an insensitive, rushed dentist, you may have had pain from his "shot," or perhaps were worked on with no anesthesia. Your good or bad past experiences will influence your degree of anxiety or relaxation.

Another factor that will either put you at ease or make you more nervous is the atmosphere in the dentist's reception room (waiting room). A quiet room with subdued lighting, pleasant colors, and perhaps soft background music, will go far to ease jangled nerves.

Promptness in seeing you will also help. Most people magnify their fears to a degree much greater than the actual experience warrants. If you are made to wait more than a few minutes, you will probably experience frustration, anger, and increased tension and anxiety. The more extensive the procedure to be performed on you that day, the more likely this is to occur. So, if you are nervous, tell the secretary you'll be there early or on time, and that you don't want to wait around for the doctor because it makes you nervous. She'll understand, and you'll feel better and more relaxed when you're taken right away.

Now let's get down to the nitty-gritty. Just what are you anxious about or afraid of? If you're like most people, thoughts like the following may run through your head:

1. Fear of the unknown: What is the dentist going to do? How will he do it? Will I have any permanent damage or esthetic deformity?
2. Will it hurt?
3. Will I gag, or swallow water, an instrument, or material, and choke?
4. Will the dentist let me rest and take a break?
5. How soon will it be over with? Will I get restless sitting still for so long?
6. How much will it hurt later, when I get home?
7. Will the dentist criticize me for not having been in for so long, for neglecting my mouth, for eating the wrong foods?
8. Will I be able to talk to the dentist or make him stop working if I get anxious?

All these are valid, important questions, which should be discussed with your dentist before he works on you, so that you do trust him and he knows your concerns.

Of all patients' fears, pain is the one most frequently expressed. Associated with pain is the feeling about getting a "shot" (needle). Since most dental procedures do stimulate nerves, and induce feelings of pressure or pain, the dental profession has long realized the need to anesthetize or numb the involved area. Simple procedures such as examinations, "cleanings," and scalings usually do not require anesthesia. But since more extensive dentistry may, let's examine the origins of the fear of pain and needles.

Most people are afraid of needles for valid reasons. They do hurt. When you were vaccinated as a child, a doctor or nurse may have surprised and hurt you. Now as an adult, when you know that you'll need a "shot" to numb you, you stiffen up with major anxiety about the forthcoming procedure. Perfectly normal and natural.

But has the dental experience with shots been made any easier for you in the past few years? The answer is yes. A humanistic dentist can help you have a more pleasant experience with several new approaches:

First, if you are apprehensive, he will let you tell him why. He wants to know what you have experienced in the past, in order to know how best to approach your fears. By talking with him, and establishing a trust and confidence in him, you will reduce your own anxiety level to some degree. He will explain to you that he has several methods of helping you with your fear of pain—and fear of any dental procedure. He will try to make it easier for you in terms of your time, length of appointments, cost, and choices of treatment; and will generally allow free communication to permit a lowering of tension.

If you are extremely anxious, he may begin by suggesting that one hour before your appointment you take 5 mg of Valium, or 200 to 400 mg of meprobamate, which he will prescribe for you. This will reduce your generalized tension, and as you become more relaxed, your interpretation of any stimulus at the dentist's hands as threatening or hurtful will be reduced. Not everyone needs a tranquilizer, but for those with very high anxiety levels, it is useful.

Another aid the dentist has, which you may already have experienced, is nitrous oxide (N_2O). This is also known as "laughing gas," and has been considered extremely safe for many, many years. It is used in combination with oxygen (O_2), in varying ratios. A minimum level of oxygen is required in all recently manufactured machines. In fact, if the oxygen begins to run low, the nitrous oxide automatically is reduced, so that the ratio can never be altered to where it might do damage.

What nitrous oxide does for you is most interesting. It has the capacity to alter your perception of what is happening to you. Some patients describe the feeling as similar to martinis. Others describe it as being like "grass." For most people, at the ratio level they prefer, it allows a relative state of euphoria and removal, or displacement of attention from what is actually going on. You know the dentist is working on you, but you really don't care. You may at times feel certain things, but you simply accept them as being O.K. You may hear music in the background, or from a set of earphones provided by the dentist, and the listening experience is enhanced. You are also not as aware of the passage of time as when you are fully awake.

Best of all, when the dental procedure is finished you can be returned quickly to a full state of consciousness and normality. This is done by turning off the nitrous oxide, and allowing you to breathe 100% oxygen for a few minutes. Assuming you've not taken any sedative or narcotic medication and have not been drinking alcohol prior to your dental visit, your brain rapidly clears itself of the previous analgesic effect of the nitrous oxide, and you're back to normal.

What other aspects of the dental visit can be made easier for you? After you're relaxed, or even if you don't desire any outside help, such as the tranquilizer or the nitrous oxide, your dentist has some things to help reduce the sting of the anesthetic needle.

He will paint a paste or salve on the mucous membrane of the mouth, in the area he intends to anesthetize. Within a few seconds, this area will become numb at the surface, where most pain receptors are. Then, when he does inject, you do not feel the penetration of the needle as much as you otherwise would.

Also, in recent years a special device has been developed that flows anesthesia under pressure into a small area. This anesthetic "blow gun" has a spring-loaded action, and forces the anesthesia into the tissue with a "pop." The benefit to you is that you barely feel the anesthesia enter with the aid of this jet-propulsion anesthetic, yet when your dentist next goes in with the needle for your deeper anesthesia, you hardly feel that. This air-pressure type of anesthesia is particularly helpful on the palate, where the firm tissue does not distend as easily as does the mucosa in the rest of your mouth.

Most anesthetics for the upper jaw are given in the fold of your gum mucosa, about one-half inch to three-quarters inch above your gum line. They have to be given individually, above each tooth, if the dentist is only working on that tooth. But for larger areas, or more extensive procedures involving gum and bone, it may be necessary to numb several teeth and the surrounding gum and bone. It is for this type of procedure that the anesthetic jet, in combination with an injection, is particularly useful. If your dentist warms the cartridge before anesthetizing you with a needle, that will greatly reduce the pain that "shots" cause. Likewise, if he injects slowly, it will greatly reduce the pain.

In addition, your dentist can help you by first giving you a "block." That is an injection used to numb a nerve trunk before it branches extensively. A block is particularly necessary in the lower jaw, because the bone is very thick in the rear areas and one can only anesthetize the molars and second bicuspid easily by using a block. From the middle of the lower jaw forward, it becomes possible to anesthetize by "infiltrating" (injecting some drops of anesthesia) near the root tip of the tooth. The anesthesia penetrates the more porous bone and numbs the tooth. "Infiltration" is usually the way the upper jaw is anesthetized.

Even on the upper, it is possible to have blocks given in several areas to start the numbness. By doing this, and waiting a few minutes, when the dentist does give you "infiltration anesthesia" over a particular tooth or teeth, you barely feel it.

This is particularly useful for longer procedures, so that the duration of the anesthesia is longer than the period during which the dentist is actively working. You are numb without having sensation return while he is still drilling or operating.

One final point about needles. The finer the tip, and the slower the dentist injects, the less likely you will be to feel what he does. The more tense and anxious you are, the more likely you are to feel the shot. So help him and yourself by using one of the aids previously described. Or, if you're not overly anxious while he injects, just breathe deeply and slowly through your nose while concentrating on some other very interesting area of your life. Place your mind elsewhere while your dentist injects. The entire procedure only takes a few seconds and, if you can cooperate, it'll be over faster than you can imagine.

The Last Resort

If, after all that has been described, you are still so afraid of going to the dentist that you'd almost rather lose your teeth, there is still one other approach you should be aware of.

That approach is either conscious sedation or general anesthesia. Conscious sedation is the use of drugs and agents to raise your pain threshold and achieve a certain degree of relaxation and tranquility while you are conscious. It is accomplished by intravenous or inhalation routes, or combinations of both. *Inhalation* is the use of a gas to produce some analgesia (raising of the pain threshold coupled with some sedation). When the *intravenous* route is used, it can be for either conscious sedation or general anesthesia.

At times, the condition you are suffering with may require that you be made unconscious. Examples of this would be severe infection or the need for very complicated surgery. Patients occasionally may be unable to cooperate through no fault of their own when they are conscious. For them, becoming unconscious under general anesthesia is the best approach. Lastly, for medical reasons, general anesthesia may be necessary.

You may wonder what you will experience on awakening. You may be dizzy and drowsy for about an hour. You should feel very little pain on awakening because there is still medication in your system. You will then be given additional pills, orally, to help you with any later discomfort. In addition, your wound may receive a sedative dressing or covering, which also helps provide relief.

If you do intend to have your dental work done using intravenous anesthesia (conscious or general), rememember:

1. You should not eat any foods or liquids for five hours before surgery or administration of the drugs.

2. Your dentist will review this with you and answer any other questions you may have.

3. Someone must meet you at the end of the visit and accompany you home.

Although dental pain and your fears are very real, the various approaches described above should go a long way toward making you comfortable, and allowing you to have the necessary dental care to help you keep your teeth.

FIFTEEN

Dental Emergencies and
Special Situations

WHAT IS AN EMERGENCY? If you are alarmed about something occurring in your mouth, causing you severe pain, swelling, or bleeding; or if you have broken a tooth, lost a bridge, or had anything else happen that you are upset about, and want to correct immediately, that is an emergency. It may not be a life-and-death situation, but if it is causing you immediate discomfort, pain, or embarrassment, it's important to have it attended to as soon as possible.

There are some very obvious dental problems that could cause you concern. You should know what to do if they arise. They include:

1. Bleeding that doesn't stop after dental surgery or tooth extraction
2. An accidental blow to a tooth, resulting in a chip or fracture of the tooth, or even causing it to be knocked out
3. Pain and soreness behind the last tooth, in the area where wisdom teeth normally exist
4. Toothache—severe pain, perhaps swelling, headache, and fever
5. Tender, bleeding gums, possible sore throat, possible fever, bad taste, and bad breath
6. An abscess or swelling of the gum next to a tooth, causing great pain
7. A human bite, usually resulting from a fight
8. Burned lips, tongue or palate, due to hot food; possibly with a child, a burn due to lye or acid

9. Uncontrolled oozing or bleeding from the gums

10. Small silvery-white sores, very painful, looking like little ulcers with red borders

11. Loss of a filling and immediate tooth sensitivity

12. Loss of a crown, bridge, or even a denture; loss of a tooth on a denture or partial denture

13. An orthodontic wire breaking and piercing the cheek or tongue

14. Nausea or suspected allergic reaction to medication being taken in relation to dental treatment

15. Floss caught between teeth

Let's discuss each of the above, so that you are prepared, or can refer to this chapter if the problem arises.

TRAUMA TO THE TEETH

One of the most common dental emergencies that occurs is the chipped or fractured tooth. This is more likely to happen to your child when he falls, than to you, although adults have been known to miss a step and meet with the same disastrous blow to the mouth. Adults and children also occasionally are in fights, or other accidents, any of which can result in the front of the face meeting with a rapidly moving hard object. Should this happen to you or your child, there are a few things to know.

Let's say the accident happened to the child.

Fracture of a Child's Tooth

How much of the tooth is chipped determines how rapidly you must get the child to the dentist. If just a small piece of enamel is chipped, and the tooth is not sensitive or loose, you can call the dentist, explain what happened, and get a normal appointment. But if a large piece of the tooth was broken, or you see the nerve (pink tissue at the center of the tooth), this is a true emergency. If your child is not already in pain, he's going to be. Call the dentist immediately so that he can prepare for the child; then go there right away.

The dentist will calm the child, and put a protective coating on the tooth, or, if the nerve is exposed, remove part of it and then protect the rest. He wants to save the tooth as long as possible, so that if it's a baby tooth, the permanent tooth will erupt into a normal space when this baby tooth is normally lost. If the damaged tooth is a permanent tooth, the dentist will try to protect that portion of the nerve in the root, to allow the root to finish developing. *Later on, your child will have a root canal, and a post-crown will be made.* For the moment, the tooth can be repaired and built back up with bonding techniques.

After emergency treatment, the tooth should be reexamined at regular intervals. For uncomplicated, small fractures, the dentist simply rounds off any sharp edges, protects any exposed dentine, and asks you and the child to return shortly. He then continues to test the tooth at one week, one month, three months, six months, and one year from the time of injury. He tests the tooth to see if it is still alive, because a blow to a tooth may cause the nerve to die. If after one year, the tooth responds normally to "vitality" testing (a test to see if the tooth is alive), it may be considered healthy. If this is a permanent tooth, then a semipermanent or permanent restoration is placed, depending on your child's age. If it is a baby tooth, the dentist will decide on the best way to restore it until it falls out during eruption of the permanent tooth. If the tooth is dying, it will need removal of the nerve, as described above. Then at a later date (one year), the dentist can decide what kind of permanent restoration to use. Roots should be completely formed before final restorative procedures.

Fracture of an Adult's Tooth

You might be interested to know what could be done if the damage occurs to you, with permanent teeth already in. The answer is determined by how much tooth structure chips off, and whether or not the nerve dies from the force of the blow. If the chip is just part of the enamel, your dentist can build up the corner of the tooth with bonding. If the dentine is also exposed, he can protect the dentine surface, which has millions of little fine canals (tubules) leading to the pulp. Afer sealing these tubules, the tooth can be built up with bonding. After checking the tooth at periodic intervals over a year, if there is no death of the nerve, then either your tooth can remain as is, or if you feel it's not as esthetic as you'd like, you can have a porcelain jacket made.

If the tooth is fractured, exposing the nerve, or fractured near the gum line, or even under it, as long as the root is intact (not fractured), you have an excellent chance of saving the tooth, with root canal and a post crown. When the fracture is under the gum, you may need periodontal surgery also, to expose sound tooth structure upon which your dentist can build a crown. Occasionally, traumatic fractures of the root may not work out well, even when the tooth is treated endodontically. This is particularly true of a vertical fracture. Your dentist is best able to make this decision, perhaps in conjunction with an endodontist's opinion.

What If the Entire Tooth Is Knocked Out?

If you get to the dentist within thirty minutes and have not damaged the tooth surface by handling it too much, there is a good chance of saving it by replanting the tooth. (See Chapter 10 under Implants, the section on replantation.) The most important point is to put the tooth into a clean handkerchief, wet with dilute salt water if possible (one teaspoon of salt in a glass of water would be the perfect solution to help preserve the living cells on the tooth surface). Do not handle the tooth by the root if you can help it. Get to the dentist immediately *after* phoning him first to alert him. He will then take over when you arrive and replant the tooth. He will stabilize the tooth, check it periodically, and advise you later on if further dental treatment, such as a post-crown, or joining it to its neighbors, is needed.

If it is your child's tooth that has been knocked out, call the dentist and tell him you're on the way over. Treatment of the child is different from that of the adult depending on the child's age. If the tooth is a primary (baby) tooth (child is age one to six), it will not be replanted. If it is a permanent tooth, it will be. Therefore, try to get to the office within thirty minutes if the tooth is a permanent one. If it's a baby tooth, the dentist will examine the child to see if there is any other dental damage, and decide on how to replace the missing tooth until the permanent tooth erupts. It is possible that when the permanent tooth does come in, it may be damaged in shape. There is nothing that can be done about it until the tooth comes into the mouth, so don't worry about it now. If damaged, it can always be bonded to restore shape, and later, crowned.

OTHER TRAUMATIC ACCIDENTS INVOLVING THE MOUTH

In addition to accidents involving one's own natural teeth, it is also possible that you already have dental replacements. You may be wearing a denture or a partial denture. If you drop this by accident, and it breaks, you can temporarily glue it, using an epoxy glue. You should not consider this permanent and should get to your dentist as soon as possible. Even slight irregularities in the surface of a denture can irritate tissues. If this irritation were to continue for too long a period, it could lead to permanent damage in the tissue next to the repaired area. Let your dentist repair and adjust the denture or partial denture properly.

Another type of accident that could occur to the mouth is a burn. Most commonly, a burn is minor; usually, from food that was too hot. Usually your palate or tongue is most affected. To get temporary relief while the tissues are healing, try rinsing with bicarbonate rinses made by mixing one teaspoonful of sodium bicarbonate to one glass of warm water. Let the mixture cool, and rinse with it several times a day, particularly before eating.

Chemical burns in the mouth might occur if a child accidentally gets hold of cleaning solutions or other industrial bottles or cans. Professional help should be sought immediately, but to provide temporary relief, determine whether the solution is acidic or alkaline. If acidic, rinse with bicarbonate of soda immediately. If alkaline, such as lye, rinse thoroughly with vinegar, followed by frequent rinses with water. Again, bring the child to a doctor or hospital as soon as possible.

A different type of emergency, but one requiring immediate attention, is a bite. Since most mouths are quite dirty, if your child is bitten by another child, immediately cleanse the wound with an antiseptic. Then call your pediatrician or physician, and let him examine the child. He may want to recommend an antibiotic.

Bleeding

There are several situations that might cause bleeding in your mouth. Always tell your dentist or dental surgeon prior to any surgical procedure if you have a family history or personal history of blood disorders or prolonged bleeding after cuts, if you have high blood pressure; or if you bruise very easily. Your dentist may want to do some laboratory studies, or to consult with your physician before he operates. Therefore, be thorough in the information you give him. It is best to avoid a bleeding problem, rather than treat it post-fact. Also, if you have been taking any medication, particularly aspirin or any other aspirin-containing medication, tell your dentist. These can alter your ability to clot. Lastly, if you are on anticoagulants, your dentist should be advised *before* he operates.

If you have no prior history of bleeding problems, and your dentist extracts a tooth, or does gum surgery, and you continue to bleed at home, what should you do? Do not rinse your mouth. Instead, cut up some gauze or clean wash cloths into 2″ x 2″ squares. Roll up the gauze pads into a ball, and place it over the bleeding area if it is an extraction socket. Bite down for thirty minutes. If it doesn't stop, take a wet tea-bag, and bite down for thirty minutes. If it still doesn't stop, call your dentist as an emergency, and see him immediately. Keep the area under continued pressure from the gauze ball or tea bag while travelling to his office.

If you have had periodontal surgery, and have a pack over the wound, apply pressure to the pack for thirty minutes with your fingers. The pressure should be gentle but firm and steady. You can use a gauze pad over the pack, and apply pressure through it against the pack. The gauze will sop up the excess blood. If this doesn't work, try the same procedure using a wet tea-bag for thirty minutes. If you still have no success, call your dentist or periodontist and arrange to be seen immediately.

In either case described, do not be alarmed if you do have to see the dentist. In most cases, merely placing a few sutures, and perhaps a special kind of dressing material, will be enough to stop the bleeding.

A different type of bleeding requiring immediate attention is spontaneous bleeding, particularly from the gums. If the gums bleed without your having done anything such as brushing, or biting into food, or accidentally bruising the gum, you should be examined immediately.

Wisdom-Tooth Infection

An infection in the wisdom-tooth area, also known as pericoronitis, usually develops from entrapment of food and bacteria under a gum flap. Often the wisdom tooth is not fully erupted, and the area is difficult to clean. These partially erupted teeth decay easily. To relieve the immediate pain, and perhaps the difficulty in opening your mouth, start rinsing vigorously with a 3 percent solution of hydrogen peroxide. Do this several times within a few hours. I recommend full strength for maximum results. If this bothers you when you rinse, dilute one-half and one-half with water. Keep the solution in your mouth for one minute, then empty. You will have bubbles or foam in your mouth, which you should rinse out with water. Call your dentist for an immediate appointment. This type of infection usually requires emergency care by the dentist, or it can get worse. For pain, take Tylenol, or Datril. Do not take aspirin, because the dentist may have to extract the tooth, and you don't want a bleeding problem.

Infection Following Surgery

A second type of infection you may experience is one that follows a surgical procedure done in your mouth. Signs of infection would be pain, swelling, and perhaps a feverish feeling. Swelling after surgery doesn't necessarily mean you have an infection, as some swelling is normal. But if the swelling keeps getting bigger, feels warm and firm, and is painful, call your dentist. He should see you immediately, and may either put you on an antibiotic or change the one you are using. He may have to open up and clean out your wound. He will know what to do once he sees you, so just make sure that if you are at all suspicious, you call him and see him. Do not take the attitude that it will probably get better by itself. It may, but if it doesn't, it is going to be harder to treat later. "An ounce of prevention is worth a pound of cure!"

Generalized Gum Infection

Another type of infection that may bother you is a generalized infection in your gum, called "trench mouth" or Vincent's. Symptoms include tender, bleeding gums, possibly fever, "wooden" feeling to the teeth, very foul odor on your breath, and possibly a sore throat. This infection is a particularly destructive, ulcerative form of gingivitis, in which the triangles of gum tissue between the teeth are rapidly destroyed by certain mouth bacteria that have increased in number. It may start with the gum between just a few teeth, and spread to the entire mouth.

Immediate treatment should start with the antibiotic tetracycline, as long as you are not pregnant, or allergic to it. If you are either, the next antibiotic of choice would be penicillin (If you are not allergic to it). Call your dentist immediately and try to see him as soon as possible. Ask him to prescribe the antibiotic if you can't get to him right away. Rinse your mouth every hour with either straight 3 percent hydrogen peroxide or diluted half and half with water until you can see him. Try to gently brush and floss to remove the debris collecting around the necks of the teeth, as this is where the bacteria are breeding. Don't worry about bleeding from your brushing or flossing efforts. This will stop within a few days as the gum condition improves. Get to your dentist and let him scale some of the debris. Within a few days to a week you should have had healing of the acute problem. Your dentist may see you several times during that week, and then weekly for scaling, for about a month. At the end of this period, by carefully inspecting the shape of the gum and examining for craters in the tissue between the teeth, he will determine if further gum treatment is needed to establish the proper shape to the gum tissue so that this condition is less likely to return again.

Some other hints during the acute stage: Stop smoking, stop drinking alcohol, try to eat as well as possible, and take at least one multivitamin per day plus 500 mg of vitamin C with each meal, and one before bedtime. Also try to get as much rest as possible, so your body has a chance to heal.

Gum Boil (Abscess)

An abscess or swelling in the gum tissue can be painful. It may result from an infection within the tooth itself, which means the nerve is dying or has died. The breakdown products seek to move in the path of least resistance through the bone and then through the gum. The abscess could also be caused by a trapping of food or bacterial products in the gum space we call a pocket. If the entrance to the pocket at the gum margin closes tightly around an area of heavy breakdown, then the toxins and breakdown products accumulate and, through pressure, may try to expand through the gum wall. Again, you may have pain with the swelling.

In both cases, you should call your dentist, tell him of your emergency, and try to be seen right away. You might ask him to call your pharmacy to prescribe a pain killer, which you will need. Temporarily, take Tylenol or Datril or, if you have nothing else, aspirin, and go to your dentist.

If for some reason you are not within reach of a dentist, you might try the following to relieve the pain temporarily (remember, this should only be done if the abscess is soft and seems to be coming to a head, like a pimple): Sterilize a needle in the blue part of a flame from the gas burner on your stove, holding the needle with a tweezer so as not to burn your finger. When it is red hot, remove it and cool it in alcohol, or let it cool by itself. Now, under a good light and looking at the area in a mirror, pierce the abscess for about one eighth inch. Gently squeeze the surrounding tissues and try to milk out any pus, or blood mixed with pus. The abscess should now be reduced in size. Do this only for temporary relief if you cannot get to a dentist right away. It is strictly a temporary measure. If you are not successful the first few times you try, do not continue. Go to a local hospital and let them get a dentist if you can't locate your own. A dentist must determine the cause of the abscess, and treat the tooth, or gum pocket, if the tooth is worth saving.

Viral Outbreaks With Mouth Sores

Another type of infection that might seem to be an emergency is a viral outbreak in your child's mouth, though it could happen in an adult. The first such attack usually does occur during childhood. There may be sores all over the mouth, sore throat, difficulty in swallowing, and possibly fever. The gums may bleed, the tongue may be bright red. Mouth odor is strong and the lymph glands may be swollen. This frequently occurs after an upper respiratory infection. Such viruses are most common in the spring and fall of the year. Call your physician and let him examine the child and advise you.

In post-childhood years, there are two other types of sores that may prove painful. One is called "herpes" and is caused by a recurrent attack of the herpes simplex virus. It is seen most often on the lip, and usually has a crusted, slightly bloody appearance. It has been associated with exposure to the sun, as well as being a local manifestation of a virus in your system. One often experiences a cold just before or after such a "cold sore." It goes away without treatment, usually in one to two weeks.

The second type of sores, canker sores, are also known as aphthous lesions. They are very painful, can occur anywhere in the mouth, and are thought to be allergy related. There has been some feeling that there may be a genetic predisposition. They have been associated with the menstrual cycle, anxiety, emotional trauma, and allergy to citric fruits. The sores look like small ulcers, yellowish-white in color, with reddish borders. The central portion may also have a silvery-whitish look to it. They last for one week to ten days. Healing is usually complete in two weeks. Call your dentist if you or your child is quite bothered by the sores. There is no specific treatment, but covering the sores with denture adhesive cream or paste seems to give them a chance to heal. Lots of rest, good, nourishing food, and the use of a multivitamin with breakfast, with dinner, and supplementary dosages of 500 mg of vitamin C with each meal and one before bedtime, should increase your general resistance and healing ability.

Pain

TOOTHACHE   There are many different causes of pain in the mouth, but certainly the most common is that of a toothache. Your home emergency approach would be to locate the tooth causing the pain, if you can. See if any of your teeth has a hole in it, or if you have lost a filling. If you can find the tooth, then placing a small cotton ball saturated with oil of cloves (from the pharmacy) into the hole in the tooth will give you temporary relief. If your tooth is tender to touch, but has no hole or lost filling, you may have an infection in the nerve. If the tooth is loose, you may have the beginning of a periodontal abscess. In any case, do not place an aspirin on the gum next to the tooth. You will burn the tissue and get an "aspirin burn." Stay away from hot or cold food or drink, and from sweets. Call your dentist immediately and get an emergency appointment. He will X-ray the tooth and treat the problem if the tooth can be saved. If he wants to pull the tooth, ask him why you can't have root canal done. He may have excellent reasons for extracting the tooth, but if he can save it, ask him to try. If he seems not to support his reasons for extraction very well, ask him to put in a temporary sedative dressing, like zinc-oxide-eugenol cement, and then get a second opinion from an endodontist.

Pain Following Tooth Extraction (Dry Socket).

An uncomplicated tooth extraction usually produces very little pain. Wisdom teeth, if impacted (buried partly or completely in the jawbone), may produce more pain during healing, but the pain usually diminishes as the days go by following the extraction. Occasionally one day or several days after an extraction, whether it was an easy or difficult procedure, you may experience pain that is quite intense and doesn't seem to get better. This could be pain from an infection. But there is another cause of pain, without an infection. That is the loss of the blood clot in the socket. Normally, the clot should be organizing and joining in the healing process. If the clot is lost, then the socket bone is bare, and no healing can occur until the bone lining the socket is undermined and removed by the cells of the surrounding bone. This can be a slow, painful process, and you may not get relief for up to two weeks. You should see your dentist as often as he suggests, and he may place medication in the socket to help comfort the area while healing occurs. He will give you the necessary prescriptions for pain killers during that period.

Pain from a Dental Procedure

You may experience pain from any dental procedure, whether on a tooth or on your tissue or bone. It is always best to call your dentist when this occurs, describe to him what it feels like, when the pain started, and whether it's increasing. He will then advise you as to what steps to take, and whether he wishes to change any of his earlier instructions.

Sudden Pain from Biting Down on a Hard Object

You may have cracked a tooth. Call your dentist immediately. He can check for a fracture with an X ray, and with a fiber-optic light. If he cannot tell for sure and you have no further pain, he may just ask you to wait a few days and see if any symptoms of a dying nerve develop. If pain is still present, then your dentist or an endodontist should decide whether root-canal treatment is indicated. The fracture may have sheared in such a way as not to involve the nerve, or it may have involved the nerve. If the fracture is vertical, the tooth will probably be lost. Only your dentist can advise you after considering all the possibilities.

OTHER EMERGENCIES

Loss of a Filling, Onlay, or Crown

If you are in your home town, call your dentist immediately. You should not go around with the inside of the tooth exposed to saliva and bacteria, even if the tooth is not sensitive. (Many times, it will be sensitive.) If you cannot get to your dentist within one or two days, go immediately to a pharmacy and get some zinc oxide powder and eugenol oil (one ounce each). On a nonabsorbent piece of paper, at home, mix the powder and small amounts of the liquid to a putty consistency. With your finger, place it in the hole in the tooth where the filling once was. Take a damp piece of cotton and tap in the white putty. Even a crown that has fallen off can be rece-mented this way, after removing all the old cement, but take the extra step of mixing in some vaseline to thin out the material, and then replace the crown. As soon as possible, get to your dentist so that he can attend to the real problem. For example, you may have decay under the filling. Don't delay seeing the dentist just because you've successfully handled the emergency. You may wind up losing the tooth. If a temporarily placed plastic crown or bridge loosens and comes out, the easiest way to replace it overnight until you see the dentist is with vaseline. Overload the cap or caps and replace them on the tooth stumps. There should be enough of a hydraulic seal to permit retention of the temporary crown until you see your dentist. Here again you should call him immediately and get the earliest possible appointment. Under no circumstances should the prepared tooth stumps be left bathing in saliva.

Dental Floss Caught Between Your Teeth

Try to work some waxed dental floss between the contact area of the two teeth until it's down under the contact (for lower teeth) or above the contact (for upper teeth). Then pass the floss outwards. If you try this twice, and still haven't been successful, call your dentist and see him. He will examine and remove the trapped floss. Don't ignore the problem, as it might cause a gum infection.

Local Allergies

On rare occasions, a patient is allergic to ingredients placed in the mouth, such as toothpaste, mouthwash, periodontal dressing, or sometimes dental materials like the various plastics used today. If the gum is red, irritated, doesn't seem to heal, and no other cause can be found, allergy should be considered, and the ingredients or materials eliminated one by one.

Problems from Braces

This is quite common with children, and even adults.

If a band or plastic bracket loosens, try to detach it without disturbing the main wire. If the band or bracket is connected, and is very irritating, you may have to disconnect it. You can use a cuticle cutter or cuticle scissors to do this. Only cut the thin wire ligature; not the main archwire. Call the dentist or orthodontist for an immediate appointment.

If the main arch wire breaks, and is sticking into the tongue, cheek, or lips, try to bend it in so it doesn't stick into the tissues. If you can't, cut it with the cuticle cutters so it will not irritate the tissues. Call the dentist or orthodontist and have a new one made.

If small fine wires between teeth loosen, try to bend them in temporarily. If you are unsuccessful, snip them off with cuticle scissors. Call the dentist or orthodontist and make an appointment.

With sore cheeks, lips, or tongue, locate the sharp or irritating part of the bracket and try to cover it with wax or chewing gum. Call the dentist or orthodontist, and let him smooth off the material causing the problem.

With broken hooks, call the dentist or orthodontist immediately, and do not wear any elastics in any other part of the mouth until he sees you.

Cheekbiting

If you are tense, or have generalized anxiety or hostility, this may manifest itself when you are sleeping, or even when you are awake. One of the ways you may express tension is by clenching or grinding your teeth. When people rub the teeth of their lower jaw against the teeth of their upper jaw, with no food present, it is called bruxing. Many people do this at night when they sleep. They may "brux," chew or even gnash their teeth. If you are doing this, you may be biting your cheek or lip. Normally, it will heal in a few days, if you don't keep chewing on that area. You should ask your dentist to help you in several ways. He can check the relationship of the bite, and see if there are any irregularities on the teeth surfaces that are contributing to your bruxing habit. If so, he can eliminate these. He also may find that in the cheek area you keep chewing, you have a sharp cusp, or an incorrect relationship of teeth. Again he can correct this. Last, he may suggest that you wear a Hawley-type appliance, or a night guard, to help break the habit and permit him to check your bite even more precisely.

You yourself can help by examining your life-style and relationships, to see what areas are tension-producing. Try to eliminate those areas or find other ways to release the tension so as to increase your general relaxation. This will reduce your tendencies to brux, or cheekbite.

SIXTEEN

Dental Insurance: What You Should Know About It

ALTHOUGH NEARLY EVERYONE recognizes the need for dental treatment, it is too often put off because of the cost. Aware of this factor, many corporations, unions, welfare funds, and welfare plans have provided their employees with group dental benefits. They often do this with the help of an insurance broker specializing in dental coverage. Dental benefits seem to be growing as estimates for the number of Americans provided with group dental insurance exceed well over sixty million people.* Conversely, individual dental insurance is very rarely offered because of the very expensive rates needed to spread the financial risk to the insurance carrier.

TOTAL COVERAGE VS. CO-INSURANCE (PARTIAL COVERAGE)

Just because an employer provides an employee and his family with dental insurance doesn't mean that the employee-patient will not have any financial obligation. The concept behind most dental insurance is to assist you in paying for part of your bill so that you are able to have more complete care. The idea is not for your employer, insurance company, or union to give you a "free ride." Since somewhere along the line, somebody's budget must pay for the dentist's

---

* M. and E. Denholtz, *How To Save Your Teeth and Your Money*, New York: Van Nostrand Reinhold Co., 1977.

time, materials, and overhead, the idea of sharing some costs, but not totally paying for everything, has become a fringe benefit of many employee groups.

Unions and employers sometimes provide dental benefits, at no cost, but with a reduction of the number of services covered. In periodontics, some closed panel* fees are so low as to make it impossible for the dentist to treat the condition. Frequently not included in the coverage is a disease control program. This unfortunately means more continued breakdown, and higher costs ultimately to the group paying for the insurance. Those plans offering periodontal care without plaque control are particularly disturbing, since it has been shown that gingivitis and periodontal disease are plaque-related conditions. Frequently, because of budget limitations and poor advice to the purchaser regarding disease prevention, the patient on limited benefit plans gets caught in the repair—breakdown—repair cycle. Groups buying low-cost insurance feel that some dental care for their employee/member is better than no dental care. It is true that repair care does help the employee to some degree, particularly in replacing teeth and filling cavities, but it is stop-gap dentistry, which in the long run will encourage further loss of teeth.

UNDERSTANDING AND USING YOUR DENTAL INSURANCE

Assuming that you have some form of dental coverage, how do you use it? There is more involved than just filling in the group insurance number, member's date of birth, social security number, and sex. To save you time, let's examine some of the basic areas.

There are several people involved in providing you with dental care, and it is most important that we clarify each of the relationships involved. You have a therapeutic and financial relationship with your dentist. You also have a relationship with your employer. Your employer (or union) has a relationship with an insurance car-

---

* A closed panel means that in order for the patient to get dental care at no cost, he must go to a dentist designated by the union as a "cooperating dentist."

rier. Your union may also be self-insured. The dentist does not have any relationship with an insurance carrier, your employer, or your union.

Most dentists contract directly with you for their services. Your financial responsibility is to them. You pay them according to the arrangements you make with them. They fill out the proper sections of the insurance forms, and when the carrier determines your benefit payment, it is sent directly to you unless assigned to the dentist.

To help you understand what financial benefits you might receive from the insurance carrier, a brief discussion of terms would be very helpful. Basically, there are two types of dental insurance:

> 1. Table of allowances (scheduled allowances)
> 2. Usual, customary, and reasonable fee (non-scheduled allowances)—abbreviated UCR from here on.

"Table of allowances" means that there is a scheduled or fixed benefit (allowance) for each dental procedure covered. The insurance company may pay 100, 90, 75 percent, or some percentage of that schedule based on the contract selected by your employer or union. For example, the plan may allow $150 for a veneer crown. It may have a deductible, and only pay the applicable percentage on the remaining balance. The allowable benefit used as a base may not be the same fee your dentist charges. It may be lower.

The second type of plan, UCR, pays a percentage of your dentist's fee. It is determined by the customary range of fees for most dentists in that geographical area at that time for that service, and then paying a percentage of the fee. If the fee charged by your dentist is above the covered charge, as determined by the carrier, you may receive benefits less than anticipated. There could also be a deductible in a UCR plan.

There are several likely questions that you may ask yourself. Let us go over some of the most common of these, so that you can apply the answers to your own situation.

How Can I Find Out If I Have Dental Insurance?

If you work for a company, ask the person who hired you. If there is a personnel director, check with him. By law, if your employer provides group health benefits, you must be given a booklet or summary plan description, and be allowed access to the master contract. If you're a union member, ask your shop steward or union secretary.

What Is the Usual Course of Events When You Hand the Dentist Your Insurance Form?

When the dentist or his staff member receives the dental form (which in the majority of offices comes from the patient and not from the doctor), he first checks to make sure that you have filled in all pertinent information. Such items as your name, group number, birth date, company name and address, whether or not you are covered by another plan, and various other particulars should be filled out by you. Then, depending on your plan requirements, the dentist may fill in a proposed treatment plan listing the services with standard codes provided by the American Dental Association.

The dentist at this point puts a date next to the examination visit and X rays (if indeed they are the only services performed to date). He then submits the form as a treatment plan pre-estimate, keeping a copy in your chart. Treatment plans including X rays and pre-estimates (predeterminations, and pre-authorizations) are usually requested for treatment cost over $100.00, over $200.00, or for certain specialty services. When all your dental work is completed, he will send a second form (the dentist's statement of actual services) to the carrier. After several days to several weeks, the treatment plan is returned with the estimate of coverage for the services to be performed. The doctor fills in the date of each service as it is performed, and at the completion of treatment signs the form and returns it to the carrier. If the plan does not require a pretreatment estimate, the doctor sends in a form for the treatment after it is completed. At times, if several procedures are scheduled over an extended period of time, the doctor may send in a form periodically, as opposed to sending in one form at completion of all treatment. The insurance company processes the form and either you or the dentist is sent a check based on the benefits already determined.

*What Kind of Dental Services Are Usually Covered
in a Dental Plan?*

Covered dental services may include:

1. Oral examinations (including diagnosis, X rays, and treatment)
2. Emergency palliative treatment
3. Extractions
4. Root-canal therapy
5. Fillings (amalgams and composites)
6. Cleanings
7. Periodontal treatments
8. Full and partial removable dentures
9. Bridgework and crowns
10. Oral surgery
11. Orthodontics

Of course most dental plans are different. Plans may list each of the above services in a more detailed manner, allowing certain services and excluding others. For example, one policy may, under periodontal surgery, cover only gingivectomies, while another policy may pay for gingivectomies, osseous (bone) surgery, bone grafts, and free soft-tissue grafts.

Under bridgework and crowns, different plans may cover different types of bridgework, and may provide payment for only certain kinds of material (for example, gold or porcelain). In most cases, the insurance company will not cover dental services done for cosmetic purposes. If your dental carrier rejects your bridgework or crowns, when they absolutely were done to replace dentistry that was failing, to repair decay and restore function or provide periodontal support for weak teeth, make sure that your dentist supports the dental health reasons for your treatment, and states in writing to the insurance company that the work was not done for cosmetic reasons.

What Dental Services Are Sometimes Covered by Medical Plans?

In some cases, such surgical procedures as periodontal surgery or oral surgery are covered by medical plans. When the patient submits the regular dental form, sometimes the carrier will either send the patient or doctor a letter stating that only certain of the procedures listed will be covered by the *dental plan*. The doctor will then have to submit another form for the other services to a *medical* division, which may be part of a separate insurance carrier. Before the regular claim is submitted, try to find out if the surgery will be covered by a medical plan. If so, the medical form can be submitted on completion of the surgical procedure.

Before you decide that you "don't have any insurance" to cover your dental needs, check with either your personnel advisor or insurance agent as to what is, and what is not, included in your medical policy.

Some medical plans will cover periodontal surgery or oral extractions only if performed in a hospital. Unfortunately, most practitioners do not have access to hospital beds for these services. In addition, many hospital operating rooms are not well equipped for periodontal surgery procedures. Thus we find two subtle ways of discouraging utilization of supposedly covered services. You may desire treatment, yet if you can't get your work done in a hospital by the dentist of your choice, you ultimately either don't get it done or you pay totally to have it done privately in the dental office. So although your policy says that you are covered for periodontal surgery, it greatly restricts your ability to receive the benefits of your coverage. Speak to your employer or health services director to get you a better policy the next time they review your group coverage.

Who Determines What Services Are Covered?

Determination of services to be covered is based on a contractual arrangement between the group or company purchasing the coverage and the carrier. The funds available for coverage may determine the extent and mix of the benefits, as well as the limitations.

Why Do Some Insurance Companies Agree to Pay Only a Certain Amount for Each Covered Service?

This occurs because the plan may have been based on the employer or union's budget. Whether they choose a "table of allowances" or a "UCR" type of policy, it still is geared to anticipated utilization by the group members. Since the paying group can only afford a limited amount, the group limits its financial liability by defining what will be covered and what the limits of coverage will be. The idea of insurance is to give you some financial help, but not to cover all your dental costs.

By limiting the covered services and the benefit, the group is able to provide for the total membership and not be overly burdened financially. The money you actually spend, if any, for your dental care, then, is the difference between the dentist's charge minus the insurance benefit. That still allows you to have more dental treatment than if you had no insurance, assuming you are on a fixed financial budget.

What Do Deductibles Mean to the Patient?

The deductible is the amount that you must pay before the plan pays for dental treatment. In some plans, a separate deductible applies to the employee and to each of his dependents. In other policies, a maximum may be placed on the total deductible for the family during the calendar year. Not all insurance policies have deductibles, or the deductibles may apply only to certain benefits. For example, it may not apply to "prevention" or diagnostic services.

It is important to note, when scheduling your dental treatment over a period of time—for example, November through March—that you may be charged with two deductibles if your plan includes a calendar-year deductible. In most dental plans, if you incur dental charges in the last three months of a calendar year, they will also apply to your deductible for the following year. You should determine whether your deductible is a one-time charge or an annual charge.

What Are Calendar-Year Limitations?

If your plan talks about calendar-year limitations, it means that not more than the calendar-year maximum will be payable under the plan for all dental expenses incurred in that calendar year. It is important to note whether or not your plan has a calendar-year maximum before you begin your dental work. Let's say that your plan has a calendar-year maximum of $1,000 and your total proposed dental treatment is $2,200. You and your dentist can then divide your work, if dentally feasible, over a two-year period.

What Is Meant by "Coordination of Benefits"?

Coordinated benefits occur when both the husband and wife are covered by insurance. In California, about 15 percent of patients have dual coverage.* Dual coverage may involve the same carrier or two different ones, depending on where the husband and wife work. The husband's insurance covers everyone in the family first, except the wife. This is the primary policy. Whatever portion of the dentist's bill is not covered by the husband's insurance is covered by the wife's insurance, but not to exceed the cost of care. The wife's insurance covers her first, and whatever is not paid is covered by her husband's insurance. His policy for her is a secondary coverage. If your children are being treated, the father's policy covers first and the mother's second.

Who Receives the Insurance Benefit?

Although most plans pay the patient directly, the patient may fill in a section assigning benefits directly to the dentist. It is the dentist's prerogative to accept or not to accept assignments. Some dentists establish a policy from the beginning of treatment that they will or will not accept assignments. Others may decide after the pre-estimate is established, and then have the patient assign the benefit directly to the dentist.

What Can You Do If You Are Not Satisfied With the Benefit You Receive?

First, reread your schedule of benefits. If you feel that you're right, call the insurance carrier and explain where you feel the error

* Denholtz, op. cit.

was made. If the carrier disagrees with you, and explains its interpretation to you, and you still feel you're right, have him request an opinion from an independent dental consultant. Also speak to your employer representative in charge of health benefits. And you might call the dental association and ask its advice on how to deal with the insurance carrier, or the insurance broker who advised your employer and helped select the coverage. As a last resort, you can call the state commissioner of insurance.

Why Don't Most Insurance Policies Cover Prevention Programs?

Although dental hygiene instruction (plaque-control instructions for bacterial removal) is considered important by many dentists, (and has been shown to be crucial in preventing long term breakdown), insurance companies are not yet convinced that it is possible to alter human behavior over a reasonably long period of time regarding dental disease control. Some of the companies also feel that it has not been possible to measure quantitatively how much benefit is produced for a given group of people who are instructed in plaque control, how long the benefit lasts, how frequently review sessions are needed, and so on. Given limited funds for dental coverage, the funds are currently directed at choosing policies to cover the repair of past neglect and breakdown, but not the prevention of future breakdown. I personally feel that this is a narrow and unenlightened view of the nature of dental disease, and how best to control it, help the public, and reduce long-term costs. Although resistance to inclusion of prevention coverage is slowly giving way, you, the consumer, can change coverage faster if you express a desire for dental disease-control programs as a covered benefit.

If good criteria were established for disease-control programs, with independent (or even insurance carrier) monitoring on a random basis, then patients could get coverage for prevention, because it would be worth it for the employer to buy that coverage. His long-term premium costs would most likely go down, as his covered employees would have less dental breakdown. Though I grant this to be an assumption, I feel that it is a very valid one. Proof of the merit of this approach is that Lindhe, et. al. have clearly shown that properly educated and monitored groups of patients can experience tremendous benefits from plaque control, including retention of teeth with very weakened bone support.* Many researchers have shown that without plaque control, dental and periodontal destruction continues.

What Objections Do Dentists Have About Insurance Coverage As It Is Now Offered?

The most common objection is that patients expect the insurance to pay for all costs, and are surprised and disappointed when they only get partial payment. As a patient, you may want to blame the dental office for not filling out the forms correctly. The problem here is that you, the patient, must study your own eligibility and benefits, as listed in your benefits booklet, and see what your coverage is.

A second objection to insurance company policy sometimes has to do with the financial award for the recommended work. The dentist can't help but object to the intrusion on the part of the third party regarding how much money will be allowed for different procedures. Although this monitor may work to the patient's benefit by preventing overtreatment, it may force you as the patient to accept a lesser quality of service. This happens when the policy will not pay for the service that your dentist recommended, and without insurance coverage to help you, you can't afford the dentist's fee. Frequently the allowances for coverage are not only grossly inadequate but are geared to services which are now obsolete. Periodontists, for example, infrequently do gingivectomies today, yet many benefit tables list "Gingivectomy . . . $— per quadrant." Today, flaps (with or without bone surgery) are the treatment of choice for moderate periodontal disease by most periodontists, yet I have had clerks refuse to authorize benefits to my patients if the form was written up that way, rather than with the code for gingivectomy. It would help if the American Dental Association were to have very frequent reviews of procedural terminology and coding so it in turn could advise the insurance companies.

Where there is disagreement over what an insurance company

* Lindhe, *Journal of Periodontology,* April 1979.

will pay for treatment, and what the dentist feels is proper treatment, then an independent third party, consisting of some appointed members of the dental society and/or the dental universities in the area, should help decide on which treatment plan is better. This is called peer review.

The problem of what services are covered and how well they are done seems to exist with many of the union plans I have seen. Sometimes the problem stems from the coverage being very limited, and the benefits being terribly low and unrealistic in today's marketplace. One finds that young dentists and specialists are hired in certain situations to treat the union employees at facilities, and are paid either a salary or percentage of what they produce. As soon as they are able to establish their private practice, they leave. As with some of the advertising centers, it becomes difficult to assure continuity with the dentist who did the original work. If covered benefits were stronger, union patients might have the choice between more complete care or going to a private dentist. Also, dentists that did want to work for such a facility, with better pay and fringe benefits, would earn enough to make it desirable to stay, and with greater coverage the dentist would feel more professional satisfaction and pride in what he would do for his patients. To change this situation, I believe that there should be at least a periodic review of allowance schedules, perhaps every three years, of both procedures offered and payments, in order to keep pace with inflation. I also feel that those plans with limited coverage because of budget restrictions are the plans most in need of preventive programs to reduce the rate of disease progression.

Can Insurance Companies Request Your Records

Yes. There is a section on the insurance form where the patient authorizes release of X rays and any other information that the insurance company may need in evaluating the claim.

What Are HMOs?

HMO stands for "health maintainance organization." "An HMO has been defined as a complete health system offering comprehensive health services and treatment to an enrolled population on a prepaid capitational basis." * Its broad purpose is to provide comprehensive care on a reimbursement basis in a way that creates economy in health care delivery. The cost is negotiated, based on the selected amount of health care to be received.

The basic concept of the HMO (a "capitation" plan) is that eligible people or families contract to pay a certain amount per person (per capita), which provides them with predetermined health-care services at regular intervals. This is in contrast to a "fee for service," which is the usual private care method. With "fee for service" you pay each time you see your doctor or dentist for the particular service (or treatment) rendered. Under a dental HMO, most dental care would be rendered without additional expense.

HMOs have been growing since the early 1970s and continue to grow. Today there are hundreds of such plans. What are their benefits?

Benefits of an HMO can include lower dental costs, as in a group practice. Because treatment of the individual is separated from payment, it is felt that there can be greater emphasis on disease prevention, eventually leading to less continuing disease, and therefore lower cost to maintain health for each participating plan member. Patients might avail themselves of dental care, especially preventive education, when they know they are not being charged for it. They also could have more frequent checkups, and not worry about the costs of each visit.

What Are Delta Dental Plans?

Delta dental plans are nonprofit dental service corporations. They were formed by organized dentistry to compete against commercial carriers. No outside insurance carrier is involved. As of 1977, according to Denholtz, the Delta system covered eleven million people.

Your own dentist, if participating in a Delta plan, can make his recommendations to you. Predetermination may be needed. If there

---

* Jerge, Charles R., et al., *Group Practice and the Future of Dental Care* (Philadelphia: Lea & Febiger, 1974), p. 18.

is any disagreement regarding the treatment plan, your dentist can request further evaluation through peer review. Here, a group of dentists will examine the dental situation and report on their findings.

Is Dental Insurance Really a Help For the Patient?

Generally, yes. In its present form, it helps solve immediate problems. Toothaches, cavities, infections, replacements for missing teeth are all very important services. More people are now seeking dental care and are going to the dentist more frequently. With more emphasis on root-canal therapy and periodontics, more teeth are being saved.

The major shortcomings are that frequently there is no benefit given for preventive measures, dietary instruction, plaque-control instruction, polishing of fillings, and so on. There should be a way to extend benefits based on a merit system. If you eat correctly, brush, and floss, your rate of dental breakdown should be less. There are ways of testing the patient's knowledge and effectiveness, and ways to evaluate rate of formation of new decay or periodontal disease activity (such as the phase microscope). If the patients do well, and indeed show little or no new disease over a period of time, they should be rewarded with more comprehensive dental benefits for themselves or their family, or the same dental coverage at lower premiums to their employers.

If you believe, as I do, that prevention is important, let your voice be heard. Make your feelings known to your employer or union officials regarding preventive care. If enough people want coverage, ways will be devised to offer it.

Your Dental Future
and the Future of Dentistry

NOW THAT YOU'VE FINISHED this book, you know what it takes to save your teeth or your children's teeth. You know about plaque, bacteria, diet, fluorides, and what good dentistry consists of. You know what to do if you have missing teeth or diseased gums, and how to improve your esthetics. You know that dentistry does not have to be as painful today as it has been in the past. You've learned that you can keep annual dental costs very low once your mouth has been brought back to a good state of health, if you practice daily plaque control and avoid refined carbohydrates.

So far, you're in pretty good shape if you've learned everything in the book. But what does the future hold? Is it possible that some day there will never be any dental disease? No cavities, no gum disease, no missing teeth? Believe it or not, this is possible, though it may take a hundred years to get there. What new events may occur in your lifetime?

I'm going to present some new developments and concepts that may be available, or are about to be released, to you as a patient. In addition, I'm going to speculate on the most likely and/or needed breakthroughs. Who knows? You may be inspired to invent one of the concepts that I envision.

Peri-Press is an existing improvement in anesthesia that permits the dentist to anesthetize a tooth that still has feeling after conventional anesthesia has been given. It is almost foolproof and should help the dentist eliminate incomplete anesthesia. It is a very fine needle that anesthetizes the periodontal membrane under very high pressure. It is now available. I foresee an improvement in this area of anesthesia in which finer and finer needles will be used with more effective anesthetic fluids, so that injections will not be felt very much and the fluids will reach and numb the nerves more quickly.

I foresee some sort of "cap" or hat, worn or attached to the head (as with biofeedback "leads"), which so pleasantly distracts the patient's attention that he pays no attention to the anesthetic needle as the shot is given. This device may or may not be accompanied by music.

In orthodontics, I see greater popularization of team approach— oral surgeon plus orthodontist—to move teeth more rapidly where the malocclusion is very bad. I see greater use of plastic brackets for esthetics. I just heard announced on the radio (July 14, 1979) that an orthodontist in California has invented brackets that permit tooth movement from the inside (tongue side) rather than the outside (face side) of the tooth. This will dramatically increase the acceptance of orthodontics by people who would like to improve their appearance but haven't wanted to bother because of brackets and/or bands showing on their front teeth.

In the field of tooth implants, glass and various ceramics, as well as other organic compounds, are being tested for biocompatibility with body tissues. At some point in time, it will be possible to implant a single artificial tooth into a hole drilled in the bone to receive it. The tooth surface will permit a true fusion or connection to the surrounding bone. The material that the tooth is made of will permit some deflection under pressure, and yet be able to return to its original shape when the pressure is released. It will have "memory." It will not be brittle or fracture easily. It will be sold in kits to dentists, and will come in various sizes and colors.

There is currently a report that such a plastic compound has been invented by a German research group. The material is reported to be biologically compatible with bone. The shaped implant is tapped into a hole prepared by the dentist. The implant itself has holes in it that bone grows into, thus anchoring the implant. The new implant is described as being bioreactive, meaning that its surface bonds chemically with bone. After three months, the patient returns to the dentist for quick and painless fitting of the crown portion of the artificial tooth onto the implant. The research team feels that this technique will replace dentures, and other removable appliances, as long as there is enough bone to support the implant.

In the field of periodontics, I see a much more specific approach to treating people by identifying the organisms in their mouths that are causing the problem. With identification, very highly specific antibiotics or chemicals might be used to interfere with the life cycles of those bacteria. In addition, in time, a vaccine should be developed to help the body build antibodies to several of the most offensive bacteria.

I also anticipate plaque solvents that industry will develop to prevent plaque from forming, or to slow down its formation. It may be possible to apply some long-lasting surface agent, either at the dental office, or in toothpaste, that will retard plaque.

I see the public being very heavily educated in the use of floss and of soft-nylon brushing into the gum space. Particular focus will be aimed at the school-age population.

I also see greater dietary instruction being given, and a shift by more educated people away from refined carbohydrates and back to a more natural diet. I see dentists learning to recognize gingivitis and periodontal disease earlier, and therefore treating people at earlier stages of the disease.

I see periodontal disease being thought of as a bacterial infection which can return even after treatment. Patients, therefore, should be continually monitored with the phase microscope to see if the wrong bacteria are again overgrowing. If so, immediate re-treatment and re-education will commence. Use of the phase microscope will increase dramatically. Today, only a small number of offices use it.

All of the above will certainly reduce the degree of periodontal disease, and bring more and more people under treatment who have suffered damage to gum and bone.

In the area of treatment, sooner or later we will have a material which can be used to fill in bony defects around teeth, and perhaps even build up support around a tooth that has lost bone. For this to occur, we will have to solve the problem of the diseased surface of the root. It will have to be decontaminated and able to fuse with a biocompatible material.

In prosthodontics, I see major changes because of new tooth-replacement techniques. There will be greater use of periodontics and orthodontics, and less reliance on capping and splinting to hold together a damaged mouth with lost teeth and lost periodontal structure. For those patients who already have capping, which has worn out and needs replacement, I see tremendous technological improvements in both esthetics and preservation of the gum and bone.

I see more conservation of tooth structure and greater emphasis being placed on occlusion. There will be improvements in filling materials and much greater use of "bonding" for esthetics, instead of capping.

In addition, I know of exciting efforts being made to permit replacement of some missing bicuspid and first molar teeth with extremely inexpensive but strong permanent replacements. It will be done with a special cast splint anchored to one or more rear teeth and one or more front teeth. As this technique comes to fruition because of much lower costs, there will be much less dependency on cast crowns and bridges and greater conservation of tooth structure. The saving for the public will be tremendous. Dentists will buy the cast splints in kits adaptable to any mouth.

In root-canal treatment, at some point in time, there will be a way to first seal the apex (tip of the root) and then fill the canal with a material that expands to create a firm fit or bond to the tooth. We are very close to that now, with a dental material that has recently been marketed. There may be a strong yet simple way to incorporate a post into the tooth and then "bond" a cap to the tooth and post.

Oral surgeons, in addition to increasing involvement with orthodontists, may get more involved with cosmetic facial surgery. Except for wisdom teeth, I see a decreasing number of tooth extractions, as time goes by, and the concepts of disease prevention and bacterial control sink in.

Pedodontics (children's dentistry) will play an increasing role in the life of many people. As more knowledge is gained about decay and nutrition, it will be the family dentist who is interested in children, as well as the pedodontist, who will guide the health of the children worldwide. As they make their presence felt, there should be less disease, and also a contribution, by those interested in stopping disease early, to public health dentistry. This means community education, rather than just individual education.

In the field of adult dental coverage, there will be more and better care made available through various dental plans and third-party coverage.

You can see that many interesting new directions are possible and probable. Your dental experiences should get easier, and your children's lifetime needs should be much less costly and dentally time consuming than yours. Everyone's esthetics can be improved, and one's teeth will indeed be helped to last a lifetime.

Where to Purchase Your Supplies

NOW THAT WE'VE DISCUSSED the various ways of maintaining optimum dental health, here are the addresses of companies where you can buy oral hygiene aids to help you in your home dental maintenance. Small or individual purchases should be made at your local pharmacy or supermarket. Large orders may be placed directly with the manufacturer.

Toothbrushes

MANUAL The following toothbrushes are representative of the soft nylon, rounded bristle tips that are most recommended for brushing in the gum space:

Reach toothbrush (Johnson & Johnson). Particularly good for small mouths and difficult-to-reach areas like molar teeth and the inside surfaces of lower front teeth.
Py-co-pay Softex. Conventional design but has benefit of rubber tip on handle if you prefer "rubber-tipping" the gum triangle between your teeth to the wooden interdental stimulators.
"G.U.M." brush (Butler).
"Oral B." "20" for small mouths or children, "40" for adults.
"Angle" brush (Squibb).

All of the above, as well as other brands, should be obtainable at your local drugstore. Remember, all toothbrushes, especially the soft ones, wear out fairly quickly. Examine the bristles once a month and, at the end of approximately three months, replace the brush if the bristles look worn.

ELECTRIC Individual toothbrushes can be obtained at drug or department stores. Quantity orders can be filled from:

Braun North America
Prudential Tower Building
Boston, MA 02199

Dominion Electric Corporation
150 Elm Street
Mansfield, OH 44902

General Electric Company
Bridgeport, CT 06602

Gillette Research Institute
Prudential Tower Building
Boston, MA 02199

Hoover Company
101 East Maple Street
North Canton, OH 44220

Pennerest 1353A
J.C. Penny Company, Inc.
1301 Avenue of the Americas
New York, NY 10019

Presto TB3
National Presto Industries, Inc.
Eau Claire, WI 54701

Ronson Corporation
Woodbridge, NJ 07095

Shavex Corporation of America
Elk Grove, Illinois; and
1801 North Central Park Avenue
Chicago, IL 60647

Sona Stream Corporation
P.O. Box 536
Peotone, IL 60468

Sunbeam Corporation
5400 West Roosevelt Road
Chicago, IL 60650

Wards Signature 14484
Montgomery Ward & Company
619 West Chicago Avenue
Chicago, IL 60607

The most important point about the electric toothbrush is that the bristles should be soft nylon, rounded tip, so that they can be placed within the gum space. A short back-and-forth motion by the brush head is better than an arcuate motion.

Dental Floss: The Most Important Aid in Plaque Removal

Johnson & Johnson Dental Floss
Johnson & Johnson
Box 308
Cherry Hill, NJ 08034
Makes waxed and unwaxed floss.

John O. Butler Company
540 North Lake Shore Drive
Chicago, IL 60611

Floss Aid, Inc.
P.O. Box 624
Santa Clara, CA 95052

Personal Dental Products Service
3714 East Indian School Road
Phoenix, AZ 85018

This is an unusual company for the individual, as it is geared to service small orders for all dental supply needs. This includes brushes, floss, floss holders, staining tablets and solutions, interdental stimulators, bridge threaders, and so on. Write to them for an order form and a product list.

P.O.H. Unwaxed Floss
Oral Health Products
P.O. Box 45623
Tulsa, OK 74145
Products from this company sold only to professionals.

Disclosing Solutions and Tablets

In order for you to best maintain healthy teeth and gums, it is necessary to know where plaque-forming trouble spots are in your mouth. Disclosing solutions and tablets will aid you in actually seeing the plaque.

You can obtain these items from your drugstore for small orders, or from:

Personal Dental Products Service
3714 East Indian School Road
Phoenix, AZ 85018

For larger orders:

Control Disclosing Solution
Dental Control Products, Inc.
Upper Montclair, NJ 07043

Red-Cote Tablets and Solution
John O. Butler Company
540 North Lake Shore Drive
Chicago, IL 60611

Plak-Chek
Clairol
345 Park Avenue
New York, NY 10022

Premier Dental Products Company
1010 Arch Street
Philadelphia, PA 19107

The Lorvic Corporation
8810 Frost Avenue
St. Louis, MO 63134

X-Pose Tablets
Proctor and Gamble Company
P.O. Box 599
Cincinnati, OH 45201

Water Irrigators

Another useful instrument in good dental health is the oral irrigating device. This instrument shoots a steady stream of water into the mouth; along with brushing, it helps to remove debris from the teeth and gums. It is not intended as a substitute for brushing. These irrigation devices, commonly known as water piks, may be found at your local drugstore, department store, or discount center.

Aqua Pulse AP-2
General Electric Company
Bridgeport, CT 06602

Assist-Dent
Clairol
345 Park Avenue
New York, NY 10022

Chic Dental Spray Company
526 Cherry Lane
Floral Park, NY 11001

Dent-O-Jet
Westminster Industries, Inc.
167 East 56th Street
New York, NY 10022

Dent-O-Pulse
Division of Troy Industries
135 Marbledale Road
Tuckahoe, NY 10707

Hydro-Gene Oral Water Spray
John O. Butler Products
540 North Lake Shore Drive
Chicago, IL 60611

Hydro Manufacturing Company
16661 Ventura Boulevard
Encino, CA 91316

Pulsar
American Sun Mark Company
P.O. Box 1330
Danbury, CT 06810

Readi-Jet II
Parke Davis & Company
Detroit, MI 48232

Turbobrush Water Pulse
Products Design and Development
Company
2 Lillian Road
P.O. Box 949
Madison, WI 53701

Water Pik
Aqua Tec Corporation
1730 East Prospect Street
Fort Collins, CO 80521

*Interdental Stimulators, Massagers,
Bridge Threaders and Personal Mouth
Mirrors*

To reach areas between the teeth
and at the neck of the teeth, the following are very useful:
Perio-Aid: Individually, order from:

Personal Dental Products Service
3714 East Indian School Road
Phoenix, Ariz. 85018

Your local drug store may carry some
of the products listed below. For large
quantities:

Perio-Aid
Marquis Dental Manufacturing
Company
2005 East 17th Avenue
Denver, CO 80206

Interdental Massage Point and
Handles
Clean-Be-Tween-Toothbrush
Company
16553 Fielding
P.O. Box 4913
Detroit, MI 48219

Lactona Stimulator Handles
and Tips
Lactona Products Division
Warner-Lambert Pharmaceutical
Company
Red Lion and Academy Roads
Philadelphia, PA 19114

Pick-A-Dent Corporation
1068 Mission Street
San Francisco, CA 94101

Proxabrush
John O. Butler Company
540 North Lake Shore Drive
Chicago, IL 60611
and
Crescent Perio Spiral Brush
Crescent Dental Manufacturing
Company
7750 West 47th Street
Lyons, IL 60534

Stim-U-Dents are used only on the
outside surface of the teeth. They differ
from stimulators primarily in that they
are made of wood. You can find them
at most drug stores.
For larger orders:

Stim-U-dent, Inc.
14035 Woodrow Wilson
Detroit, MI 48238

A mouth mirror will enable you to
look into the back of your mouth and
to look at your teeth from different
angles, thus enabling you to cleanse
your mouth more efficiently. Mouth
mirrors, manufactured by John O. Butler Company and the Floxite Company, Inc., may be obtained at:

Personal Dental Products Service
3714 East Indian School Road
Phoenix, AZ 85018

Other manufacturers for large orders, besides the Butler Company include:

Plastic Mirrors
Sam Dixon
18434 Tapham Street
Tarzana, CA 91356

Sherman Specialty Company
Merrick, NY 11566

Union Broach Company, Inc.
36-40 37th Street
Long Island City, NY 11101

Floxite Company, Inc.
Box 1094
Niagara Falls, NY 14303

Semantodontics
P.O. Box 15668
Phoenix, AZ 85060

It is most important that you be able to floss even if you have bridgework. Bacteria are still accumulating in the gum spaces between your teeth. To help you, *bridge threaders* may be purchased at your drugstore.
Large orders may be obtained from:

#840 EEZ-THRU
John O. Butler Company
540 North Lake Shore Drive
Chicago, IL 60611

BRIDGEAID
Floss Aid Corporation
P.O. Box 624
Santa Clara, CA 95052

If you are a teacher or would like your child's teacher to educate his or her students in tooth care, perhaps you should provide the names of the following companies where oral hygiene kits may be obtained. These kits contain various educational materials as well as the oral hygiene aids that would be useful in classroom demonstrations. The kits are manufactured by:

American Dental Association
Bureau of Audiovisual Service
211 East Chicago Avenue
Chicago, IL 60611

Block Drug Company, Inc.
Jersey City, NJ 07302
Toothpastes for Sensitive Teeth

Sensodyne
Thermodent
Protect

The above should be available at your pharmacy or large discount center (health aids section).

Bibliography

1. *Proper Examination*

Bucholz, R.E. "Histologic-Radiographic Relation of Proximal Surface Carious Lesions." *Journal of Preventive Dentistry.* Vol. 4, no. 6 (November-December 1977).

Melton, John C. "How to Picture Your Patient's Periodontal Status by Recording Four Signs of Periodontal Disease." *General Dentistry.* Vol. 25, no. 6 (November-December 1977).

Sabes, William R., and Blozis, George G. "The Clinical Laboratory: What It Means to You and Your Patients." *Journal of the American Society for Preventive Dentistry.* Vol. 3, no. 6 (November-December 1973).

2. *Periodontal Diagnosis*

Hurt, William C. "Periodontal Disease—1977—A Status Report." *Journal of Periodontology,* 48 (September 1977): 533-539.

Simpson, John, Miester, Frank, Jr., and Gerstein, Harold. "Differential Diagnosis of the Endodontic-Periodontic Lesion." *Journal of the Western Society of Periodontology, Periodontal Abstracts.* Vol. 27, no. 1 (1979).

3. *Orthodontics*

Chaconas, Spiro J. "Preventive Orthodontics: When and Why." *Journal of Preventive Dentistry.* Vol. 5, no. 3 (May-June 1978).

Freeman, Julian D., "Preventive and Interceptive Orthodontics: A Critical Review and the Results of a Clinical Study." *Journal of Preventive Dentistry.* Vol. 4, no. 5 (September-October 1977).

Olson, R. E. et. al. "Orthosurgical Teamwork." *Journal of the American Dental Association* 90 (May 1975).

Silverstein, Alvin, and Silverstein, Virginia B. *So You're Getting Braces: A Guide to Orthodontics*. Philadelphia and New York: J. B. Lippincott Co., 1978.

Sim, Joseph M. "Interceptive Orthodontic Treatment of Malocclusions in Younger Children." *Journal of the American Society for Preventive Dentistry*, Vol. 6, no. 5 (October 1976).

4. Oral Surgery

Bowers, G. M. "Study of the Width of Attached Gingiva." *Journal of Periodontology* 34: (May 1963): 201–9.

Kruger. *Textbook of Oral Surgery*. St. Louis: The C.V. Mosby Co. 1959.

Lindhe, J., and Nyman, S. "The Effect of Plaque Control and Surgical Pocket Elimination on the Establishment and Maintenance of Periodontal Health. A Longitudinal Study of Periodontal Therapy in Cases of Advanced Disease." *Journal of Clinical Periodontology* 2 (2) (April 1975) 67–79.

McCarthy, Frank M., *Emergencies in Dental Practice*. 2nd ed. Philadelphia: W. B. Saunders Co., 1972.

Ochsenbein, C., "Current Status of Osseous Surgery." *Journal of Periodontology* 48: 377–86.

Ramfjord, S. P., et al. "A Longitudinal Study of Periodontal Therapy." *Journal of Periodontology* 44 (February 1973): 66–7.

Ramfjord, S. P. "Present Status of the Modified Widman Flap Procedure." *Journal of Periodontology*, 48 (September 1977): 558–564.

Shluger, S. "Osseous Resection: A Basic Principle in Periodontal Surgery." *O.O.O.* 2 (1949): 316.

5. Endodontics

Sommer, Ostrander, and Crowley. *Clinical Endodontics*. 2nd ed. Philadelphia and London: W. B. Saunders Co., 1961.

6. Pedodontics

Moss, Stephen J. *Your Child's Teeth*. Boston: Houghton Mifflin Co., 1977.

Nowak, Arthur J. "Prevention of Dental Disease from Nine Months in Utero to Eruption of First Tooth." *Journal of the American Society for Preventive Dentistry*. Vol. 6, no. 5 (October 1976).

7. Implant

"Implantologist." *The International Journal of Oral Implantology*, Vol. 1, no. 3 (August 1978).

Linkow, L. J., and Chercheve, R. *Theories and Techniques of Oral Implantology*. Vols. 1, 2. C. V. Mosby Co., 1970.

Schnitman, Paul A., and Shulman, Leonard B. "Recommendations of the Consensus Development Conference on Dental Implants." *Journal of the American Dental Association.* Vol. 98 (March 1979).

8. *Emergencies*

Srawder, Kenneth D. "Traumatic Injuries to Teeth of Children." *Journal of Preventive Dentistry.* Vol. 3, no. 6 (November-December 1976).

9. *Pain and Anxiety*

Aspects of Anxiety. Philadelphia and New York: J. B. Lippincott Co., 1965.
Bennett, Richard C. *Monheim's Local Anesthesia and Pain Control in Dental Practice.* 6th ed. St. Louis: The C. V. Mosby Co., 1978.
Chasens, A. L., and Kaslick, Ralph S. "Mechanisms of Pain and Sensitivity in the Teeth and Supporting Tissues." Workshop, Fairleigh Dickinson University School of Dentistry; American Academy of Oral Medicine, 1974.
Hassett, James. "Why Dentists Are a Pain in the Mind." *Psychology Today,* Vol. 11, no. 8 (January 1978).
Trieger, Norman. "Pain Control." *Quintessence,* 1974.
Weisenberg, Matisyohu. *Pain: Clinical and Experimental Perspectives.* St. Louis: The C. V. Mosby Co., 1975.

10. *Insurance*

Jerge, Charles R., et al. *Group Practice and the Future of Dental Care.* Philadelphia: Lea and Febiger, 1974.
"Third Party Insurance: Guidelines for Bringing Preventive Dentistry Under Contract." *Journal of the American Society for Preventive Dentistry.* (November-December 1971).

11. *X Rays*

Alcox, Ray W., and Jameson, Wayne R. "Patient Exposures From Intraoral Radiographic Examinations." *Journal of the American Dental Association* 88 (March 1974) 568–579.
Bushong, Stewart C. "Radiation Exposure in Our Daily Lives." *The Physics Teacher* (March 1977) 135–144.
Gibbs, Julian S. "Preventive Dental Radiology." *Journal of the American Society for Preventive Dentistry* (January-February 1976).
Goldman, Henry, and Stallard R. "Limitations of the Radiograph in the Diagnosis of Osseous Defects in Periodontal Disease." *Journal of Periodontology,* Vol. 44, no. 10 (October 1973).
HEW Publication (FDA) 77-8021, *Eighth Annual National Conference on Radiation Control. Radiation Benefits and Risks: Facts, Issues, and Options* (May 2–7, 1976).

Lilienthal, Bernard. "Radiation Reduction in Dental Radiology." *Journal of the American Society for Preventive Dentistry* (January-February 1976).

Little, John B., and Williams, Jerry R. *Handbook of Physiology—Reactions to Environmental Agents.* Ch. 8, "Effects of Ionizing Radiation on Mammalian Cells."

NCRP Report No. 45, *Natural Background Radiation in the United States Recommendations of the National Council on Radiation Protection and Measurements.* National Council on Radiation Protection and Measurements, Washington, D.C. 20014 (November 15, 1975).

Prichard, John F., "The Roentgenographic Depiction of Periodontal Disease." *Journal of the American Society for Preventive Dentistry* (March-April 1973).

Updegrave, W. J. "Dental Radiography With The Versatile Intraoral Positioner System." *Journal of Preventive Dentistry.* Vol. 4, no. 3 (May-June 1977).

Webster, E. W., and Merrill, O. E. "Radiation Hazards II Measurements of Gonadal Dose in Radiographic Examinations." *New England Journal of Medicine* 257 (October 24, 1957): 811–819.

12. Nutrition

Abrahamson, E. M., and Pezet, A. W. *Body, Mind, and Sugar.* New York: Holt, Rinehart, and Winston, 1951.

Alban, Arthur L. "Dental Office Nutrition Counseling." *Journal of the American Society for Preventive Dentistry* (May-June 1975).

Atkins, Robert C. *Dr. Atkins' Super Energy Diet.* New York: Crown Publishers, Inc., 1977.

Brennan, R. O., and Mulligan, W. C. *Nutrigenetics.* New York: M. Evans and Co., 1975.

Burton, Benjamin T. *Human Nutrition* (formerly *The Heinz Handbook of Nutrition*). 3d ed. New York: McGraw-Hill Book Company, 1976.

Clark, J. W., Cheraskin, E., and Ringsdorf, William, Jr. *Diet and the Periodontal Patient.* Springfield, Ill.: Thomas, 1970.

Clark, W. James. *Clinical Dentistry.* Vol. 1, ch. 22. New York: Harper & Row, 1977.

Dufty, William. *Sugar Blues.* New York: Chilton Book Co., 1975.

Hazen, Stanley P. "Diet, Nutrition, and Periodontal Disease." American Society for Preventive Dentistry Workshop, Aug. 4–7, 1974. Published by the American Society for Preventive Dentistry.

Hoffer, A., and Walker, M. *Orthomolecular Nutrition.* New Canaan, Conn.: Keats Publishing, Inc., 1978.

Hrachovec, Josef P. *Keeping Young and Living Longer.* Los Angeles: Sherbourne Press, Inc., 1972.

Kreitzman, Stephen N. "New Perspectives on Diet and Dental Caries." *Journal of Preventive Dentistry,* Vol. 5, no. 1 (January-February 1978).

Labuza, Theodore P. *The Nutrition Crisis.* St. Paul, Minn., New York, N.Y.: West Publishing Co., 1975.

Leonard, Jon N., Hofer, J. L., and Pritikin, N. *Live Longer Now.* New York: Charter Books, 1974.

Masters, Donald M., and Lewis, Howard. "The Sour Side of Sugar." *Journal of the American Society for Preventive Dentistry* (January-February 1975).

Morehouse, Lawrence E. *Total Fitness in 30 Minutes A Week.* New York: Simon and Schuster, 1975.

Muller, Alice, and Allen, Gene. *Sprouts, How To Grow and Eat Them.* Printed by Moore's Graphic Arts, 256 Potrero Street, Santa Cruz, California 95060.

Nizel, Abraham E. "The Practice of Nutrition in Dental Caries Prevention." *Journal of the American Society for Preventive Dentistry* (January-February 1975).

Null, Gary. *Body Pollution.* New York: Arco Publishing, 1973.

Oliver, Martha H. *Add A Few Sprouts to Eat Better for Less Money.* New Canaan, Conn.: Keats Publishing Co., 1975.

Passwater, Richard. *Supernutrition for Healthy Hearts.* New York: Jove/Harcourt Brace Jovanovich, 1978.

Pauling, Linus. *Vitamin C and the Common Cold.* San Francisco: W. H. Freeman and Co., 1970.

Shaw, James H., et al. *Textbook of Oral Biology.* Ch. 11, "Nutrition." Philadelphia: W. B. Saunders Co., 1978.

Stone, Irwin. *The Healing Factor,* New York: Grosset & Dunlap, 1972.

Williams, Roger J. *Nutrition Against Disease.* Belmont, Cal.: Fearon-Pitman, 1971.

Yudkin, J. *Sweet and Dangerous.* New York: Wyden, Inc., 1972.

13. *Sealants*

Cons, Nahaur C., et al. "Adhesive Sealant Clinical Trial: Results of a Three-Year Study in a Fluoridated Area." *Journal of Preventive Dentistry.* Vol. 3, no. 3 (May-June 1976).

Gwinnett, John A. "The Scientific Basis of the Sealant Procedure." *Journal of Preventive Dentistry,* Vol. 3, no. 2 (March-April 1976).

Handelman, Stanley L. "Microbiologic Aspects of Sealing Carious Lesions." *Journal of Preventive Dentistry.* Vol. 3, no. 2 (March-April 1976).

Horowitz, H. S., Heifetz, S. B., and Poulsen, S. "Adhesive Sealant Clinical Trial: An Overview of Results After Four Years in Kalispell, Montana." *Journal of Preventive Dentistry.* Vol. 3, no. 3 (May-June 1976).

Rudolph, Jerome J., Phillips, Ralph W., and Swartz, Marjorie L. "In Vitro Assessment of Microleakage of Pit and Fissure Sealants." *Journal of Prosthetic Dentistry.* Vol. 32, no. 1 (July 1979).

Stiles, H. M., et al. "Adhesive Sealant Clinical Trial: Comparative Results of Application by a Dentist or Dental Auxiliaries." *Journal of Preventive Dentistry.* Vol. 3, no. 3 (May-June 1976).

14.   Disease Prevention

Bakdash, Bashar M. "Patient Motivation and Education." *Clinical Preventive Dentistry.* Vol. 1, no. 2 (March-April 1979).

Caldwell, Robert C., and Stallard, Richard E. *A Textbook of Preventive Dentistry.* Philadelphia: W. B. Saunders Co., 1977.

Chambers, D. W. "Patient Susceptibility Limits to the Effectiveness of Preventive Oral Health Education." *Journal of the American Dental Association.* Vol. 95, no. 6 (December 1977).

"The Dental Clinics of North America." *Chairside Preventive Dentistry* (October 1972).

DiOrio, Louis P., and Madson, Kenneth O. "Patient Education—A Health Service for the Prevention of Dental Disease." *Journal of the American Society for Preventive Dentistry* (November-December 1971).

Donkin, R. T. "Oral Irrigation in Your Patient's Home Care Control Program." *Journal of the American Society for Preventive Dentistry* (March-April 1972).

Doyle, Walter A. "Prevention—How Much, When, Why, For Whom?" *Journal of the American Society for Preventive Dentistry,* (September-October 1973).

Glickman, Irving, Symposium on Chairside Preventive Dentistry. *The Dental Clinics of North America,* Vol. 16, no. 4, Oct. 1972, Philadelphia, W. B. Saunders Co.

Gomer, Ronald M., et al. "The Effect of Oral Rinses." *Journal of the American Society for Preventive Dentistry* (March-April 1972).

Hausman, E., and Hausmann, B., "Motivation—Key to Patient Success in Mechanical Plaque Control." *Journal of the American Dental Association* 92 (February 1976) 403–408.

Heifetz, Stanley B., et al. "Combined Anticariogenic Effect of Fluoride Gel-Trays and Fluoride Mouthwashing in an Optimally Fluoridated Community." *Clinical Preventive Dentistry.* Vol. 6, no. 1 (January-February 1979).

Jackson, David B., D.D.S., M.S. "Longitudinal Studies: What Has Been Learned about the Prevention and Treatment of Periodontal Disease," *Clinical Preventive Dentistry* Vol. 1, no. 3 (May-June 1979).

Katz, Simon, McDonald, James L., and Stookey, George K. *Preventive Dentistry in Action.* Upper Montlcair, N.J.: D.C.P. Publishing, 1976.

Kleinberg, Israel, "Prevention and Dental Caries," *Journal of Preventive Dentistry.* Vol. 5, no. 3 (May-June 1978).

Lang, Ni, et al. "Toothbrushing Frequency As It Relates to Plaque Development and Gingival Health." *Journal of Periodontology.* Vol. 44, no. 7 (July 1973).

Legler, Donald W. "Current Concepts in Clinical Preventive Dentistry—A Critical Assessment." *Journal of the American Society for Preventive Dentistry* (September-October 1972).

Mansky, Marvin. "Plaque Control for the Dentist—for the Patient." *New York State Dental Journal.* Vol. 38 (December 1972).

Marthaler, T. M. "Improved Oral Health of School Children of Sixteen Communities After Eight Years of Prevention." *III. Gingival Conditions and Calculus. Schweiz. Mschr. Aznhheilk* 86 (1976): 891–906.

Melcer, Samuel, Feldman, Stephen M. "Preventive Dentistry Teaching Methods and Improved Oral Hygiene—A Summary of Research." *Clinical Preventive Dentistry.* Vol. 6, no. 1 (January-February 1979).

Ostrom, Carl A. "Effectiveness of a Preventive Dentistry Delivery System." *Journal of the American Dental Association.* Vol. 97 (July 1978).

"Progress Against Oral-Facial Disease." *Journal of the American Dental Association.* Vol. 87, no. 5. Special Issue N.I.D.R. 25th Anniversary Conference.

Schmid, M. O., et al. "Plaque Removing Effect of a Toothbrush, Dental Floss, and a Toothpick." *Journal of Clinical Periodontology* 3 (1976): 157–165.

Shannon, I. L., and Edmonds, E. J. "Reduction of Enamel Solubility by Various Fluoride Compounds, Each Containing 1.23 Percent Fluoride." *General Dentistry, Journal of the Academy of General Dentistry.* Vol. 25, no. 5 (September-October 1977).

Silverstone, Leon M. *Preventive Dentistry,* London and Fort Lee, N.J.: Update Books, 1978.

Stanton, Gilbert, "Diet and Dental Caries." *Journal of the American Society of Periodontology* (November-December 1971).

Suomi, John D. "Prevention and Control of Periodontal Disease." *Journal of the American Dental Association.* Vol. 83 (December 1971).

Theilade, J. "Development of Bacterial Plaque in the Oral Cavity." *Journal of Clinical Periodontology* 4 (1977) 1–12.

Waerhaug, Jens. "Healing of the Dento-Epithelial Junction Following Sub-Gingival Plaque Control I, As Observed in Human Biopsy Material." *Journal of Periodontology.* Vol. 49, no. 1 (January 1978).

————————————. "Healing of the Dento-Epithelial Junction Following Sub-Gingival Plaque Control II, As Observed on Extracted Teeth." *Journal of Periodontology,* Vol. 49, no. 3 (March 1978).

Ward, Howard L., and Miller, Harold. *A Preventive Point of View.* Springfield, Ill.: Charles C. Thomas, 1978.

15.   *Etiology of Periodontal Disease*

Allison, A. C. *The Lancet,* p. 1002–1003, Nov. 1976

Baer, Paul N., and Benjamin, Sheldon D. *Periodontal Disease in Children and Adolescents.* Philadelphia and New York: J. B. Lippincott Co., 1974.

Cattoni, M., and Shannon, I. L. "Laboratory Study of Patients with Advanced Periodontal Disease." *Journal of the Western Society of Periodontology.* Vol. 24, no. 4 (Winter 1976–77).

Ceravalo, F. J., and Baumhammers, A. "Halitosis." *Journal of the Western Society of Periodontology.* Vol. 21, no. 4 (Winter 1973).

————————————, Baumhammers, A., and Robin, G. "The Odor Emitted From Dental Floss Used on Flossed Teeth and Non-Flossed Teeth For a One-

Week Time Period." *Journal of the Western Society of Periodontology*, Vol. 21, no. 4 (Winter 1973).

Diefenbach, Viron, "The Dental Plague." *Journal of the American Society for Preventive Dentistry* (October 1970).

Eastcott, A. D., and Stallard, R. E. "Sequential Changes in Developing Human Dental Plaque as Visualized by Scanning Electron Microscopy." *Journal of Periodontology*. Vol. 44, no. 4 (April 1973).

Edwards, Richard C. "Bleeding Index: A New Indicator in Personal Plaque Control." *Journal of the Society for Preventive Dentistry* (May-June 1975).

Fischman, Stuart L., et al. *Journal of Preventive Dentistry*. Vol. 2, no. 1 (January-February 1975).

Guinard, Emilio A., and Caffesse, Raoul G. "Localized Gingival Recessions: 1. Etiology and Prevalence." *Journal of the Western Society of Periodontology*. Vol. 25, no. 1 (Spring 1977).

Listgarten, M. A. "Structure of the Microbial Flora Associated With Periodontal Health and Disease in Man: A Light and Electron Microscopic Study." *Journal of Periodontology* 47 (1) (January 1976) 1–18.

Listgarten, M. A., and Hellden, L. "Relative Distribution of Bacteria at Clinically Healthy and Periodontally Diseased Sites in Humans." *Journal of Clinical Periodontology* 5 (1978): 115–132.

Loe, H., et al. "Experimental Gingivitis in Man." *Journal of Periodontology* 36 (May-June 1965): 177–87.

Mackler, B. F., et al. "Immunoglobulin-Bearing Lymphocytes and Plasma Cells in Human Periodontal Tissue." *Journal of Periodontal Research* 12 (1977): 37–45.

Marshall, H. B. "Plaque and Periodontal Disease." *New York Journal of Dentistry*. Vol. 41, no. 6 (June-July 1971).

Newman, H. N. "The Apical Border of Plaque in Chronic Inflammatory Periodontal Disease." *British Dental Journal* 141 (1976): 105.

Newman, M. G., and Socransky, S. S. "Predominant Cultivable Microbiota in Periodontitis." *Journal of Periodontal Research* 12 (2) (March 1977): 120–28.

Novaes, A. B. Jr., Rubin, M. P., and Kramer, G. M. "Proteins of the Gingival Exudate: A Review and Discussion of the Literature." *Journal of the Western Society of Periodontology, Periodontal Abstracts*. Vol. 27, no. 1 (1979).

Nolte, William A. *Oral Microbiology*. 3d ed. St. Louis: The C. V. Mosby Co., 1977.

Oshrain, H., et al. "Periodontal Status of Patients with Reduced Immunocapacity." *Journal of Periodontology*. Vol. 50, no. 4 (April 1979).

Page, Ray C., et al. "Chronic Inflammatory Gingival and Periodontal Disease." *Journal of the American Medical Association*. Vol. 240, no. 6 (11 August 1978).

Salkind, A., Osrain, H. I., and Mandel, I. D. "Bacterial Aspects of Developing Supragingival and Subgingival Plaque." *Journal of Periodontology* 42 (November 1971): 706–8.

Samant, A., et al. "Gingivitis and Periodontal Disease in Pregnancy." *Journal of Periodontology* 47 (1976): 415.

314   HOW TO SAVE YOUR TEETH

Selvig, K. A. "Attachment of Plaque and Calculus to Tooth Surfaces." *Journal of Periodontal Research* 5 (1970): 8–18.

Socransky, S. S. "Microbiology of Periodontal Disease—Present Status and Future Considerations." *Journal of Periodontology* 48 (September 1977): 497–504.

——————————. "Relationship of Bacteria to the Etiology of Periodontal Disease." *Journal of Dental Research* 49 (March-April 1970): 203–22.

16. *Epidemiology*

Marshall-Day, C. D., Stephens, R. G., and Quigley, L. F., Jr. "Periodontal Disease: Prevalence and Incidence." *Journal of Periodontology* 26 (1955): 185.

Russell, A. L. "Epidemiology of Periodontal Disease." *International Dental Journal* 17 (June 1967): 282–96.

World Health Organization. "Epidemiology, Etiology, and Prevention of Periodontal Diseases." Technical Report Series 621, World Health Organization, Geneva, 1978.

17. *Anatomy-Histology*

Scott, James Henderson, and Symons, Norman B. B. *Introduction to Dental Anatomy.* Edinburgh and London: Churchill Livingstone, 1974.

18. *Biology of the Periodontium*

Slavkin, H. C., "Toward a Cellular and Molecular Understanding of Periodontics. Cementogenis Revisited." *Journal of Periodontology* 47 (5) (May 1976): 249–55.

19. *Occlusion*

Zander, H. A. and Polson, A. M. "Present Status of Occlusion and Occlusal Therapy in Periodontics." *Journal of Periodontology* 48 (September 1977): 540–44.

20. *Periodontal Research*

Aleo, J. J., et al. "In Vitro Attachment of Human Gingival Fibroblasts to Root Surfaces." *Journal of Periodontology* 46 (November 1975): 639–45.

Alfano, Michael C. "Prospects for Improving the Prevention of Inflammatory Periodontal Disease." *Journal of Preventive Dentistry.* Vol. 5, no. 1 (January-February 1978).

Axelsson, P., and Lindhe, J. "Effect of Controlled Oral Hygiene Procedures on Caries and Periodontal Disease in Adults." *Journal of Clinical Periodontology* 5 (1978): 133–51.

—————————————. "The Effect of a Plaque Control Program on Gingivitis and Dental Caries in School Children." *Journal of Dental Restoration* 56 (1977): C142.

Becker, W., Berg, L., and Becker, B. "Untreated Periodontal Disease: A Longitudinal Study." *Journal of Periodontology.* Vol. 50, no. 5 (May 1979).

Hancock, E. B., et al. "The Relationship Between Gingival Crevicular Fluid and Gingival Inflammation: A Clinical and Histologic Study." *Journal of Periodontology.* Vol. 50, no. 1 (January 1979).

Hochberg, Joseph A. "An Interview with Dr. Sigmund S. Socransky." *Northeastern Society of Periodontists Bulletin* (April 1977).

Listgarten, M. A. "Structure of the Microbial Flora Associated with Periodontal Health and Disease in Man: A Light and Electron Microscopic Study." *Journal of Periodontology* 47 (January 1976): 1–18.

Matsson, L. "Development of Gingivitis in Preschool Children and Young Adults." *Journal of Clinical Periodontology* 5 (1978): 24–34.

Ranney, R. R. "Immunofluorescent Localization of Soluble Dental Plaque Components in Human Gingiva Affected by Periodontitis." *Journal of Periodontal Research* 13 (1978): 99–108.

Ruben, Morris P., and Shapiro, Allen. "An Analysis of Root Surface Changes in Periodontal Disease—A Review." *Journal of Periodontology.* Vol. 49, no. 2 (February 1978).

Schenkein, H. A., and Genco, R. J. "Gingival Fluid and Serum in Periodontal Diseases: I. Quantitative Study of Immunoglobulins, Complement Components, and Other Plasma Proteins. II. Evidence for Cleavage of Complement Components C_3, C_3 Proactivator (Factor B), and C_4 in Gingival Fluid." *Journal of Periodontology* 48 (1977): 772, 778.

Sidaway, D. A. "A Microbiological Study of Dental Calculus: I. The Microbial Flora of Mature Calculus; II. The Invitrocalcification of Microorganisms from Dental Calculus." *Journal of Periodontal Research* 13 (1978): 349–66.

Wilde, G., Cooper, M., and Page, R. C. "Host Tissue Response in Chronic Periodontal Disease: VI. The Role of Cell-Mediated Hypersensitivity." *Journal of Periodontal Research* 12 (1977): 179–96.

Williams, B. L., et al. "Subgingival Microflora and Periodontitis." *Journal of Periodontal Research* 11 (February 1976): 1–18.

21.   Periodontal Treatment

Becker, W., Berg L., and Becker, B. "Untreated Periodontal Disease: A Longitudinal Study." *Journal of Periodontology.* Vol. 50, no. 5 (May 1979).

Calagna, Lawrence J. "A Comprehensive Treatment Rationale Combining Prosthodontics and Periodontics." *Journal of Prosthetic Dentistry.* Vol. 30, no. 5 (November 1973).

Cohen, Charles I. "Periodontal Surgery for the Apprehensive Patient with Anesthetic Management—A Review of 150 Patients." *Journal of Periodontology.* Vol. 50, No. 1 (January 1979).

Ewen, S. J., and Gwinnett, A. J. "A Scanning Electron Microscopic Study of Teeth Following Periodontal Instrumentation." *Journal of Periodontology* 48 (1977): 2.

Goldman, Henry, and Cohen, D. Walter. *Periodontal Therapy.* 5th ed. St. Louis: The C. V. Mosby Co., 1973.

Goodman, Stephen F. "Maintenance Care: A Must in Periodontal Therapy." *New York State Dental Journal.* Vol. 44, no. 1 (January 1978).

Hamp, Sven-Erik, Nyman, Sture, and Lindhe, J. "Periodontal Treatment of Multirooted Teeth: Results After Five Years." *Journal of Clinical Periodontology* 2 (1975): 126–35.

Hirschfeld, Leonard, and Wasserman, Bernard. "A Long-Term Survey of Tooth Loss in 600 Treated Periodontal Patients." *Journal of Periodontology.* Vol. 49, no. 5 (May 1978).

Jones, William A., and O'Leary, Timothy J. "The Effectiveness of In Vivo Root Planing in Removing Bacterial Endotoxin from the Roots of Periodontally Involved Teeth." *Journal of Periodontology.* Vol. 49, no. 7 (July 1978).

Knowles, J. W., et al. "Results of Periodontal Treatment Related to Pocket Depth and Attachment Level, Eight Years." *Journal of Periodontology.* Vol. 50, no. 5 (May 1979).

Lie, T., and Meyer, K. "Calculus Removal and Loss of Tooth Substance in Response to Different Periodontal Instruments." *Journal of Clinical Periodontology* 4 (1977): 250–62.

Lindhe, Jan, and Nyman, Sture. "The Effect of Plaque Control and Surgical Pocket Elimination on the Establishment and Maintenance of Periodontal Health: A Longitudinal Study of Periodontal Therapy in Cases of Advanced Disease." *Journal of Clinical Periodontology* 2 (1975): 67–69.

Listgarten, M. A., Lindhe, J., and Hellden, L. "Effect of Tetracycline and/or Scaling on Human Periodontal Disease: Clinical, Microbiological, and Histological Observations."

Maynard, J, and Gary J.; Wilson, Richard D. K. "Physiologic Dimensions of the Periodontium Significant to the Restorative Dentist." *Journal of Periodontology.* Vol. 50, no. 4 (April 1979).

Melton, John C. "How to Picture Your Patient's Periodontal Status by Recording Four Signs of Periodontal Disease." *General Dentistry.* Vol. 25, no. 6 (November-December 1977).

Northeastern Society of Periodontists, Inc. "Guidelines for the Assessment of Clinical Quality in Periodontal Therapy and Professional Performance of Periodontal Procedures" (1978).

Nyman, Sture, Rosling, Bengt, and Lindhe, Jan. "Effect of Professional Tooth Cleaning on Healing After Periodontal Surgery." *Journal of Clinical Periodontology* 2 (1975): 80–86.

———, Lindhe, Jan, and Rosling, Bengt. "Periodontal Surgery in Plaque-Infected Dentitions." *Journal of Clinical Periodontology* 4 (1977): 240–49.

———, and Lindhe, Jan. "A Longitudinal Study of Combined Periodontal and

Prothetic Treatment of Patients with Advanced Periodontal Disease." *Journal of Periodontology*. Vol. 50, no. 4 (April 1979).

Ramfjord, S. P., et al. "Longitudinal Study of Periodontal Therapy." *Journal of Periodontology*. Vol. 44, no. 2 (February 1973).

————. "Present Status of the Modified Widman Flap Procedure." *Journal of Periodontology* 48 (1977): 558–64.

Rau, C. F. "Recognizing Early Clinical Signs of Periodontal Disease," *Quintessence Int.* 56 (1977): 51.

Rosenberg, Marvin M. and Clark, James W. "Management of Osseous Defects." *Clinical Dentistry*. Vol. 3, Ch. 10.

Rosling, B., Nyman, S., and Lindhe, J. "The Effect of Systematic Plaque Control on Bone Regeneration in Infrabony Pockets." *Journal of Clinical Periodontology* 3 (1976): 38–53.

Ross, Ira F., and Thompson, Robert M., Jr. "A Long-Term Study of Root Retention in the Treatment of Maxillary Molars with Furcation Involvement." *Journal of Periodontology*. Vol. 49, no. 5 (May 1978).

Sepe, Walter W., et al. "Clinical Evaluation of Freeze-Dried Bone Allografts in Periodontal Osseous Defects, Part II." *Journal of Periodontology*. Vol. 49, no. 1 (January 1978).

Sternberg, Victor M., and Marshall, Howard B. "Biological Basis for Placement of Crown Margins." *New York State Dental Journal*. Vol. 42 (December 1976).

Sternlicht, Harold C. "Evaluating Long-Term Periodontal Therapy—What Constitutes Success or Failure?" *Journal of Preventive Dentistry*. Vol. 2, no. 4 (July-August 1975).

The Fifth Annual USC Periodontal Symposium: Scaling and Curettage—Is It Enough? USC School of Dentistry, 26–27 January 1979.

Van Volkinburg, J. W., et al. "The Nature of Root Surfaces After Curette, Cavitron, and Alphasonic." *Journal of Periodontal Research* 11 (1976): 374–81.

Weiss, T. "Transplants and Implants in Periodontal Osseous Surgery—A Literature Review." *Acta Parodontologica*, in: Schweiz, Mtschr. Zahnheilk, 86: 103, January 1976.

Wilkinson, R., and Maybury, J. E. "Scanning Electron Microscopy of the Root Surface Following Instrumentation." *Journal of Periodontology*. Vol. 44, no. 9 (September 1973).

Zamet, J. S. "A Comparative Clinical Study of Three Periodontal Surgical Techniques." *Journal of Clinical Periodontology* 2 (1975): 87–97.

Zander, H. A., and Polson, A. "Present Status of Occlusion and Occlusal Therapy in Periodontics." *Journal of Periodontology* 48 (1977): 540.

22. Restorative Dentistry

Eames, B. Wilmer, et al. "Techniques to Improve the Seating of Castings." *Journal of the American Dental Association*. Vol. 96 (March 1978).

Goldstein, Ronald E. *Esthetics in Dentistry*. Philadelphia and New York: J. B. Lippincott Co., 1976.

Graver, Herbert T. "Restorative Dentistry Must Be Preventive Dentistry." *Journal of Preventive Dentistry.* Vol. 3, no. 5 (September-October 1976).

Ibsen, Robert L. and Neville, Kris. *Adhesive Restorative Dentistry.* Philadelphia, London, and Toronto: W. B. Saunders Co., 1974.

Luescher, Bernard, et al. "The Prevention of Microleakage and Achievement of Optimal Marginal Adaptation." *Journal of Preventive Dentistry.* Vol. 4, no. 2 (March-April 1977).

Med Com, Inc.: Esthetics 1973

Mehta, Noshir R., et al. "Stresses Caused by Occlusal Prematurities in a New Photo Elastic Model System." *Journal of the American Dental Association.* Vol. 93 (August 1976).

Noble, Warden H., Tueller, Vern M., and Douglass, Gordon D. "Margin Placement in Restorative Dentistry." *Journal of the American Society for Preventive Dentistry.* Vol. 3, no. 4 (July-August 1973).

Saltzberg, D. S., et al. "Scanning Electron Microscope Study of the Junction Between Restorations and Gingival Cavosurface Margins." *Journal of Prosthetic Dentistry.* Vol. 36, no. 5 (November 1976).

23. Restorative Factors

Karlsen, K. "Gingival Reactions to Dental Restorations." *Acta. Odont. Scand.* 28 (December 1970): 895–904.

Ricter, W. A. and Ueno, H. "Relationship of Crown Margin Placement to Gingival Inflammation." *Journal of Prosthodontic Dentistry* 30 (August 1973): 156–61.

24. Oral Hygiene

Albino, Judith E. "Evaluation of Three Approaches to Changing Dental Hygiene Behaviors." *Journal of Preventive Dentistry.* Vol. 5, no. 6 (November-December 1978).

Arnim, S. S. "Dental Irrigators for Oral Hygiene, Periodontal Therapy, and Prevention of Dental Disease." *Journal of the Tennessee Dental Association* 47 (April 1967): 63–65.

———. "Use of Disclosing Agents for Measuring Tooth Cleanliness." *Journal of Periodontology* 34 (May 1963): 245–77.

Axelsson, P. and Lindhe, J. "Effect of Controlled Oral Hygiene Procedures on Caries and Periodontal Disease in Adults." *Journal of Clinical Periodontology* 5 (1978): 133–51.

Bass, C. C. "An Effective Method of Personal Oral Hygiene." *Journal of the Louisiana State Medical Society* 106 (1954): 101.

Evans, Richard I. "Motivating Changes in Oral Hygiene Behavior: Some Social Psychological Perspectives." *Journal of Preventive Dentistry.* Vol. 5, no. 4 (July-August 1978).

Friedman, Lawrence A., and French, Christine I. "Evaluation of an Oral Hygiene

Program for Preschool Children." *Journal of Preventive Dentistry*. Vol. 5, no. 6 (November-December 1978).

Gwinnett, John A., Golub, Lorne M., and Kleinber, Israel. "The Use of Ultraviolet Photography and Crevicular Fluid Flow Rate in the Evaluation of an Amine Fluoride Dentifrice." *Journal of Preventive Dentistry*. Vol. 5, no. 6 (November-December 1978).

Lindhe, J., and Nyman, S. "The Effect of Plaque Control and Surgical Pocket Elimination on the Establishment and Maintenance of Periodontal Health. A Longitudinal Study of Periodontal Therapy in Cases of Advanced Disease." *Journal of Clinical Periodontology* 2 (2) (April 1975): 67–79.

Loe, H., and Silness, J. "Periodontal Disease in Pregnancy." *Acta Odont. Scand.* 21 (1963): 533–51.

Ripa, Louis W., Barenie, James T., and Leske, Gary S. "The Effect of Professionally Administered Biannual Prophylaxes on the Oral Hygiene, Gingival Health, and Caries Scores of School Children." *Journal of Preventive Dentistry*. Vol. 3, no. 1 (January-February 1976).

Saxer, V. P., Turconi, B., and Elsasser, Ch. "Patient Motivation with the Papillary Bleeding Index." *Journal of Preventive Dentistry*. Vol. 4, no. 4 (July-August 1977).

Suomi, John D., Leatherwood, Ernst C., and Chang, Jacqueline J. "A Follow-Up Study of Former Participants in a Controlled Oral Hygiene Study." *Journal of Periodontology*. Vol. 44, (November 1973).

———, and Doyle, Joe. "Oral Hygiene and Periodontal Disease in an Adult Population in the United States." *Journal of Periodontology*. Vol. 43, no. 11 (November 1972).

———, et al. "The Effects of Controlled Oral Hygiene Procedures on the Progression of Periodontal Disease in Adults: Results After Third and Final Year." *Journal of Periodontology*. Vol. 42, no. 3 (March 1971).

25. Fluoride

Keyes, Paul, and Englander, Harold R. "Fluoride Therapy in the Treatment of Dentomicrobial Plaque Disease." *Journal of the American Society for Preventive Dentistry* (January-February 1975).

Ripa, Louis W., Leske, Gary S., and Lowey, Warren G. "Fluoride Rinsing: A School-Based Dental Preventive Program." *Journal of Preventive Dentistry*. Vol. 4, no. 5 (September-October 1977).

Wachtel, L. W. "Topical Fluoride Controversy Symposium." *Journal of the American Society for Preventive Dentistry*. Vol. 3, no. 5 (September-October 1973).

Webster, David B., Jr., and Ringelberg, M. L. "A Sodium Fluoride Mouthrinse Program for Florida Schools." *Journal of the American Society for Preventive Dentistry* (April 1977).

Wei, Stephen H. Y., and Wefel, James S. "Topical Fluoride in Dental Practices." *Journal of Preventive Dentistry*. Vol. 4, no. 4 (July-August 1977).

26. *Lay Books*

Cranin, Norman A. *The Modern Family Guide to Dental Health*, Briarcliff Manor, N.Y.: Stein and Day, Inc., 1968.

Denholtz, M., and Denholtz, E. *How to Save Your Teeth and Your Money.* New York: Van Nostrand Reinhold Co., 1977.

Himber, J. *The Complete Family Guide to Dental Health.* New York: McGraw-Hill Book Co., 1974.

McGuire, Thomas. *The Tooth Trip.* New York: Random House, and The Bookworks, 1972.

27. *Miscellaneous*

Accepted Dental Therapeutics, 37th Edition. American Dental Association, 1977.